NOURISH
The Cancer Care Cookbook

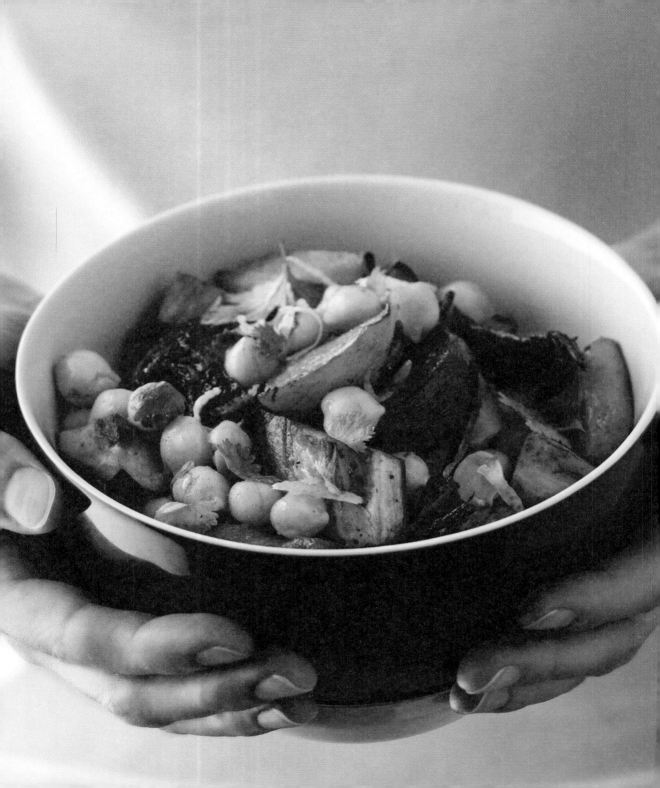

NOURISH
The Cancer Care Cookbook

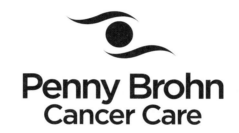

Penny Brohn
Cancer Care

with **Christine Bailey**

DUNCAN BAIRD PUBLISHERS

LONDON

NOURISH
Penny Brohn Cancer Care
with Christine Bailey

Distributed in the USA and Canada by
Sterling Publishing Co., Inc.
387 Park Avenue South
New York, NY 10016-8810

First published in the UK and USA in 2013 by
Duncan Baird Publishers, an imprint of
Watkins Publishing Limited
Sixth Floor
75 Wells Street
London W1T 3QH

A member of Osprey Group

Managing Editor: Grace Cheetham
Editor: Jan Cutler
Americanizer: Beverly LeBlanc
Managing Designer: Luana Gobbo
Production: Uzma Taj
Commissioned Photography: William Lingwood
Food Stylist: Emily Jonzen
Prop Stylist: Lucy Harvey

ISBN: 978-1-84899-084-5

10 9 8 7 6 5 4 3 2 1

Typeset in Adobe Caslon Pro
Color reproduction by XY Digital
Printed in Italy by L.e.g.o. S.p.a.

Notes on the recipes Unless otherwise stated:
• Use large eggs, medium fruit and vegetables
• Use organic ingredients, where possible
• Use meat from animals that have been grass fed
• Use organic or free-range eggs
• Use gluten-free, dairy-free and low-salt home-made stock or
  cubes or granules
• Use wild Alaskan salmon
• All-purpose and wholewheat flour should be measured
  by spooning into the cup and leveling
• 1 tsp = 5ml   1 tbsp = 15ml   1 cup = 240ml

Some recipes also include healthy alternatives. If possible, use
the following ingredients where specified: coconut oil for
cooking; nutritional yeast flakes; and raw cacao powder or cacao
nibs in place of unsweetened cocoa powder or chocolate.

The food symbols refer to the recipes only, not to any serving
suggestions. Pine nuts have been classed as nuts. Honey,
molasses, xylitol and stevia have been classed as sugars. Check
the manufacturer's labeling, because the ingredients used
in different brands vary, especially for small quantities
of ingredients such as soy and sugar, although manufacturers are
not required to detail minuscule quantities of ingredients.

Acknowledgments Penny Brohn Cancer Care would like to
thank staff: Wendy Burley, BA (Hons), DNTh, MBant, PGCert,
Lead Nutritional Therapist; Dr. Catherine Zollman, MRCP,
MRCGP, Fellow in Integrative Medicine, Lead Integrative
Doctor; Dr. Eleni Tsiompanou, MD, Diploma in History and
Philosophy of Medicine, MSc in Nutritional Medicine,
Integrative Doctor. With special thanks to funders: The Gerald
Micklem Charitable Trust, The Cyril Corden Trust, The
February Foundation, The Sir Charles Jessel Charitable Trust,
The Coutts Charitable Trust. Thank you also to the nutrition
and services teams and the chefs at Penny Brohn Cancer Care,
who contributed to the work of the cookbook, and to all those
who tested the recipes.

For information about custom editions, special sales, premium
and corporate purchases, please contact Sterling Special Sales
Department at 800-805-5489 or specialsales@sterlingpub.com.

Contents

Our Whole-Person Approach 6

**Eat Well, Live Well—Natural Foods
   & Cancer 10**
   The Link Between Diet & Cancer 12
   Our Approach to Healthy Eating 16
   The Power of Food—Where to Find the
      Nutrients You Need 24
   Managing Treatment & Side Effects 30
   Maintaining a Healthy Weight 34
   How to Eat Well 36
   Frequently Asked Questions 42
   Seven-Day Menu Plans 46

**Shakes, Juices, Smoothies &
   Breakfasts 48**

Soups & Light Dishes 66

Main Meals 92

Desserts & Baked Treats 118

**Supporting Your Body Through
   Treatment 136**
   Nausea 138
   Loss of Appetite & Weight Loss 142
   Immune System 146
   Fatigue 150
   Digestive Problems 154

Index 160

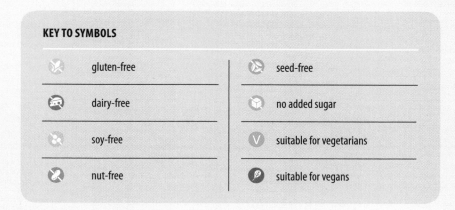

KEY TO SYMBOLS

gluten-free		seed-free	
dairy-free		no added sugar	
soy-free		suitable for vegetarians	
nut-free		suitable for vegans	

Our Whole-Person Approach

Eating well is a simple and powerful way to strengthen your body's natural defenses against cancer. We aim to help you enjoy nourishing food and a whole-person lifestyle. Our understanding is based on more than thirty years' experience of helping people to live well with the impact of cancer.

Penny Brohn Cancer Care has supported tens of thousands of people since 1980, as they take this step and make other simple lifestyle changes. Our approach, which has become known as The Bristol Approach, is a powerful combination of physical, emotional, psychological and spiritual support that is designed to help anyone affected by cancer, at any stage of the disease.

Working alongside medical treatment, our philosophy encourages people to build up their own resilience and to harness the power of their body's innate capacity to restore balance and well-being (the technical term for this is homeostasis). We are the leading United Kingdom charity working in this field.

When Penny Brohn was diagnosed with cancer in 1979 she asked, "Is there anything I can do to help increase my chances of staying well?" It set her on the path that led her, and her friend Pat Pilkington, to found the charity that is now known as Penny Brohn Cancer Care. The philosophy was to take a whole-person approach to managing cancer—and this continues to be our aim today.

Nourish is for people affected by cancer, including their family and friends—although much of the information applies to anyone, whatever their age or state of health. It is a source of recipes, inspiration and practical nutritional information that can increase your chances of staying well.

How does a whole-person approach affect cancer cells?
Cancer is a complex group of diseases. There are many different types, with numerous causes. Each cancer type can affect our bodies in a number of ways. In essence, each cancer starts life as a normal cell in which the DNA has been damaged. The

damaged cell divides rapidly, multiplying and invading areas of the body where it would not normally be found.

Cancer is often caused by free-radical damage, which creates "oxidative stress" in the body. It uses processes such as angiogenesis (page 13) to grow and spread, and can be encouraged by certain environments in the body, such as inflammation.

The good news is that your body is hard-wired to heal. Your immune system is designed to protect you from all kinds of damage and has specialized white blood cells whose job it is to detect and destroy cancer cells. How a cancer develops depends on the balance between the damaged cells and the ability of your body's immune system to detect and destroy them. Learning how to support your immune system is an essential step toward making your body a less cancer-friendly environment. This is especially important during cancer treatment, which often has the side effect of temporarily reducing immune function.

Your immune system is sensitive to changes in your physical, emotional and psychological states. There can be times when you seem to catch every cold going, especially when you've been under pressure or have been burning the candle at both ends. Now, scientists have proved that white blood cells can be activated or deactivated by chemicals produced in the body; for example, epinephrine and cortisol, which your adrenal glands make when you are stressed, are powerful immune suppressants, whereas endorphins—produced by your body when you exercise—are immune enhancers.

Fortunately, many of the things that keep your immune system working well also make you feel good, so it is a question of listening to your body and finding the right balance for you.

Eating well and exercising regularly, managing your stress and emotions, and connecting to the things and people that really matter in your life are all ways that can help increase your chances of staying well.

THE FIRST SIMPLE STEPS TOWARD A WHOLE-PERSON APPROACH

• Eat more whole foods, especially vegetables and fruit, and fewer processed foods.

• Aim to build up to doing some form of exercise for 20 minutes, five times a week.

• Identify any major sources of stress in your life and, if these can't be changed, use regular mindfulness meditation or relaxation to help minimize the effects of the stress on your health.

• Make sure you have support for expressing your emotions when you need to; for example, a cancer nurse specialist, your doctor, through counseling, a support group, friends or family, or by using an online forum or keeping a diary.

• Do at least one small thing every day that lifts your spirits or connects you to the things that matter to you.

Can changing your lifestyle really alter cancer growth?

Researchers who have studied whole-person approaches have found that when people eat more healthily, exercise more regularly and pay attention to managing their stress and emotions, their cancers can sometimes become less active and even shrink in size. Evidence confirms the benefits of such lifestyle changes and how they can increase survival in people with cancer.

These results don't in any way suggest that medical treatments are not needed —this approach can work even more effectively when combined with conventional care—but they do highlight the potential benefits of a whole-person approach for the many millions of people living with a cancer diagnosis in the world today.

You, food and *Nourish*

For many people, improving their diet is the first step toward managing their cancer, and this cookbook will help you to do that. There is more to our approach than the food you eat. The benefit you get from eating well depends on many things; if you eat meals "on the run," for example, blood flow will be diverted away from your digestive organs, so even if you eat healthily your body might not be able to use the food as well as it could, reducing some of the nutritional benefit. Similarly, if worry about your health is causing lack of sleep or arguments with your family, or if you don't exercise, the overall benefit of the good food you eat might be reduced. What is more, if you're tired, stressed or depressed, you are likely to spend less time cooking and can be more likely to reach for comfort foods instead, which tend to be high in sugar, salt and unhealthy fats—precisely the foods that undermine the body's ability to heal itself.

The intention behind *Nourish* is to help you to adopt healthy eating as a lifestyle. We take you step by step through our approach, explaining at each stage why the food combinations we suggest make a difference to the way your body is able to deal with cancer cells and cancer treatments. In The Link Between Diet & Cancer (page 12) we explain the science behind our approach and what this means for you in practical terms. In How to Eat Well (page 36) there are tips on how to plan, prepare and eat your meals in a relaxed way. There are also suggestions to help you get the most from the food you eat by making sure your digestion is working at its best.

We hope by reading and using *Nourish* you will be inspired to have fun experimenting with new ideas, new foods and new ways of eating. You'll learn how to increase your resistance to cancer and, by choosing from the many recipes we've selected, you'll make sure mealtimes become a daily opportunity to support yourself and live well.

Bon appétit!

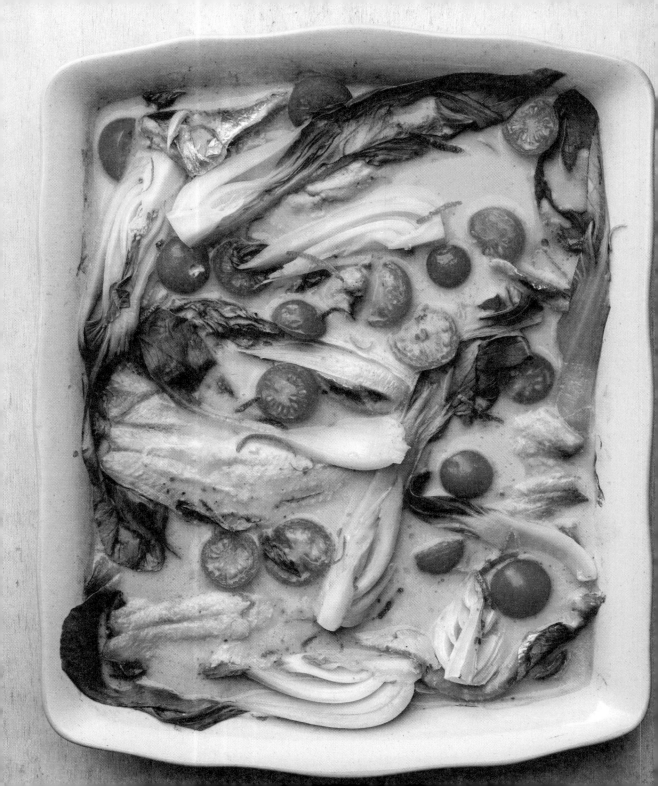

Eat Well, Live Well—
Natural Foods & Cancer

In this section we introduce you to the reasoning behind our philosophy at Penny Brohn Cancer Care, and the concepts we adopt for living well with cancer and managing any side effects you might have from treatments. You will find information on foods and nutrition and how it can support your body. We also list the beneficial properties of a variety of foods we recommend you eat often. The daily menu plans at the end of this section will help you decide which meal combinations you will enjoy, using the recipes in this book. Each day's menu focuses on providing a balance of nutrients through a wide range of wholesome foods and flavorings.

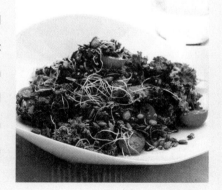

Opposite: Coconut- & Lime-Baked Sardines (page 81)
Above: Wilted Kale Salad with Toasted Seeds (page 87)

The Link Between Diet & Cancer

Cancer is on the increase, and it is estimated fifty percent of people alive today will be diagnosed with the disease in their lifetime. Experts from the World Cancer Research Fund and the American Institute for Cancer Research reviewed the evidence in 2007 and agreed diet is the single most important factor responsible for this massive rise. It is likely to be responsible for thirty-five percent of all cancers—an even greater risk than cigarette smoking. They issued clear guidelines: aim to be slim without being underweight; avoid sugary drinks; eat a variety of healthy whole foods, mainly of plant origin; eat less red and processed meats; and limit alcohol and salt intake.

To understand why diet makes such a difference, it helps to know a little about how cancer develops. Cancer takes advantage of unhealthy environments in the body and uses sophisticated processes to spread. Some of these environments and processes are explained below, as well as how good food can help to protect you.

Why avoiding inflammation is important

Persistent inflammation, swelling or redness, creates an environment that supports cancer at all stages of tumor development, so foods that help to minimize this are very important. If you include in your diet more omega-3 fatty acids (found in oily fish), but fewer omega-6 essential fatty acids (found in polyunsaturated cooking oils, such as sunflower and vegetable, and in margarines and processed foods), this helps your body to reduce any inflammation. The fiber, vitamins and other antioxidants found in fruit, vegetables and whole grains can also help to reduce inflammation. What is more, recent research shows omega-3 fatty acids might be able to boost the anticancer effect of the breast-cancer drug Tamoxifen.

On the other hand, trans-fats (found in margarines and processed foods) and too many omega-6 fatty acids can encourage inflammation. Not only do they contribute to conditions that favor cancer, but they can also contribute to heart disease, atherosclerosis, metabolic syndrome and other chronic conditions.

Beyond this, foods with a high glycemic index (GI) and glycemic load (GL) create a pro-inflammatory environment in the body. The glycemic index and glycemic load are ways of measuring how quickly the carbohydrates in food are broken down to create glucose in the blood. White bread, white rice (excluding basmati rice), most cereals and foods containing sugar are some of the foods with high GI and GL values. They all make inflammation more likely and/or more pronounced.

Most people enjoy sugar, so it can be hard to accept that it undermines health. Nevertheless, there are several links between sugar, inflammation and cancer growth (see also The Effects of Hormonal Imbalances and Insulin Resistance, page 14), which is why reducing sugar consumption is a major step toward protecting your well-being.

Vitamin D is thought to have a key role in reducing inflammation in the body. For the most part, vitamin D can be made in the body by the daily action of sunlight on the skin, without burning. Vitamin D-rich foods include oily fish, shellfish, egg yolks, mushrooms and butter.

Foods that control the growth of cancer cells

Cancer cells use angiogenesis (the creation of new blood vessels) to supply the oxygen and nutrients they need to grow. Angiogenesis is a naturally occurring process in your body, but in a cancerous situation the rate of new blood-vessel formation is abnormally rapid. Scientists have discovered natural food products that help to stop the creation of new blood vessels and are testing them for their potential therapeutic use. By including foods such as shallots, garlic, soybeans, cruciferous vegetables, citrus fruit, spices, green tea and many herbs, you benefit from their antiangiogenic properties, thereby helping to slow down the creation of the new blood vessels that help cancerous cells to grow.

Slowing down cell division

Cancer cells tend to multiply rapidly, but some foods are able to arrest their growth by interfering with the process of cell division; for example, indole-3-carbinol (I3C) stops cancer cells dividing by locking away an enzyme called elastase. I3C is found in cruciferous vegetables—eating vegetables like cabbage, cauliflower and broccoli, therefore, slows down the rate at which cancer cells multiply.

Our genes respond to our lifestyle

It is common to believe our genes determine the risk of developing cancer and it is coded into our DNA at birth. In fact, only five to ten percent of cancers are caused by hereditary factors. Studies from a relatively new branch of biology, called epigenetics, are showing how the genes we inherit are affected by lifestyle, dietary choices and events. This illustrates how genes are not always our destiny and the lifestyle choices we make can be very powerful in controlling them; a diet rich in folic acid, for example, found in green vegetables, helps to promote healthy epigenetic processes and resists the formation and spread of cancerous cells.

The effects of hormonal imbalances and insulin resistance

Cancer growth can also be stimulated by hormonal imbalances. This is more evident in hormone-sensitive cancers, such as breast and prostate cancer. Being overweight or obese increases the risk of these cancers, as well as others, including endometrial, colon, pancreatic and kidney.

Obesity also induces insulin resistance. This is where the body no longer tolerates high levels of glucose, causing insulin levels to rise. Insulin works as a growth factor for many cells, especially those in the colon. And, if these cells grow out of control, they can become cancerous. In advanced stages of cancer, insulin resistance contributes to weight loss and feeling weak.

Being a healthy weight is an important step toward protecting yourself from hormone-sensitive cancers, insulin resistance and other chronic diseases.

The damaging effects of stresses on the body

The production of free radicals is a normal chemical reaction in the body; however, we live in a world that promotes the overproduction of free radicals: smoking and drinking alcohol, as well as environmental pollution and stress, are just some of the triggers that prompt their formation. When the body is in contact with too many free radicals, it is unable to limit the cell damage they cause, and this accumulates over time. The result is known as oxidative stress, which drives cancer initiation and development. More recent studies suggest cancer cells might also deliberately create oxidative stress around them to destroy the normal cells and steal their nutrients for their own use.

Antioxidants are chemicals that "mop up" free radicals and reduce their damaging effects. The damage of free radicals in the body can be limited by including foods that are rich in antioxidants, such as vitamins C and E, and the minerals selenium and zinc. Plant foods are your first choice for these nutrients: vegetables, fruit, seeds and nuts. Zinc and selenium are also found in meat and seafood.

Our Approach to Healthy Eating

At the core of the Penny Brohn Cancer Care approach to healthy eating is the belief that foods in their most natural state are the best for you. A whole-food diet based on fresh, unprocessed foods will keep you the healthiest you can be. We recommend a diet based primarily on plant foods, vegetables and fruit, whole grains, legumes, nuts, seeds, herbs and spices. We also recommend some animal products alongside the plant foods, but in a smaller amount.

Organic or not organic?

If you can, choose organically produced foods, particularly animal products. Two good reasons to eat organic are that these foods have lower levels of potentially harmful residues and, according to scientific research, they can have higher levels of beneficial nutrients. Organic foods tend to be relatively more expensive and not as widely available, so you might want to combine organic and nonorganic foods in each meal. The most important thing is to eat a wide variety of whole foods.

Food basics in a nutshell

The principles of a cancer-preventative diet are summed up by balance, variety, color and moderation. Eat a good balance of the different food groups and vary the foods you eat from within those groups—the color of your food is a good indication of its nutritional value. The more color variety the more nutrient value.

Choosing what to put on your plate

It's possible your plate will look very different from what you have been used to. A large portion of your healthy-eating plate should be made up of vegetables and it will include some other plant foods (fruit, whole grains, legumes, nuts and seeds), too. There will be some protein, either in the form of animal products or legumes. You need protein to build and maintain every cell in your body, and protein in

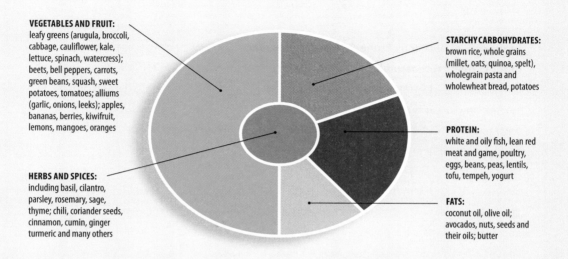

VEGETABLES AND FRUIT:
leafy greens (arugula, broccoli, cabbage, cauliflower, kale, lettuce, spinach, watercress); beets, bell peppers, carrots, green beans, squash, sweet potatoes, tomatoes; alliums (garlic, onions, leeks); apples, bananas, berries, kiwifruit, lemons, mangoes, oranges

HERBS AND SPICES:
including basil, cilantro, parsley, rosemary, sage, thyme; chili, coriander seeds, cinnamon, cumin, ginger turmeric and many others

STARCHY CARBOHYDRATES:
brown rice, whole grains (millet, oats, quinoa, spelt), wholegrain pasta and wholewheat bread, potatoes

PROTEIN:
white and oily fish, lean red meat and game, poultry, eggs, beans, peas, lentils, tofu, tempeh, yogurt

FATS:
coconut oil, olive oil; avocados, nuts, seeds and their oils; butter

your food also helps to regulate the release of sugar into your bloodstream. You also need to eat healthy fats, so they should be included on the plate, too, in the form of vegetable oils, nuts and seeds, or butter. And finally, if you add some herbs and spices to your plate, you'll boost the flavor of your food and benefit from their powerful health-enhancing properties.

There can be treats, too

Follow the healthy-eating guidelines outlined here ninety percent of the time and the odd treat won't hurt. Most people find that after eating healthy foods for a while, their tastes change, and they prefer wholesome foods. You might find your old idea of a food treat will no longer appeal in the same way.

You are in control

The simple and general guidelines in the following pages are there to help you assess your own dietary intake and judge whether you need to increase the amount you eat of some types of food and reduce others. Certain foods might be more important on some occasions, whereas others will be more appealing at other times, and you might need to adapt your meals to maintain a good balance.

Foods to eat on a daily basis

Plan to eat the following foods daily and include a wide variety of those listed in the Power of Food chart on pages 24–9.

VEGETABLES AND FRUIT   Various scientific studies have shown vegetables and fruit can help protect against cancer. They also contain compounds that support health in general, including fiber, vitamins, minerals and phyto- (plant) nutrients.

We recommend eight portions of fresh vegetables and two to three portions of fruit every day. Choose a variety of vegetables and fruit in an array of colors, to make sure you get the full range of important phytonutrients. A simple way to estimate a portion size is to work out the amount of a vegetable or fruit will fit into your cupped hand.

PROTEIN FOODS   One of the vital roles protein plays in your diet is in helping your body to repair itself. Cells can be damaged by disease, injury, surgery and even treatment, so sufficient protein from the diet is essential. Your body also needs protein to maintain a healthy immune system and to prevent infection.

We recommend some protein at each meal. On average, we recommend animal products five to six times a week—eggs or a palm-size portion of meat, poultry or fish. Animal products are good sources of protein and those we particularly recommend are white meat, lean red meat and game, fish and eggs. Ideally, use a variety of animal and vegetable proteins, because they have different properties. If you choose a vegetarian diet, however, make sure you regularly eat sources of plant protein—legumes, nuts and seeds—and high-protein grains, such as quinoa.

LEGUMES Also known as pulses, legumes include beans, lentils and peas. They have a relatively high protein content compared to other plant foods, and are also good sources of fiber, vitamins, minerals and phytonutrients, including phytoestrogens. We recommend a variety of well-cooked or sprouted legumes— sprouting enhances the nutritional benefits. Minimize beans if your digestive system is delicate.

WHOLE GRAINS Grains that are unrefined— whole grains— contain fiber, B vitamins, vitamin E and a range of minerals and essential fats.

We recommend a variety of whole grains, including quinoa, millet, barley, buckwheat and rye, as well as spelt (lower in gluten than wheat), wheat, rice and oats. If you are not eating animal products, combine grains with legumes.

HEALTHY FATS Your body requires fats to absorb some nutrients, such as the fat-soluble vitamins and minerals. They also assist brain function and improve insulin resistance. Healthy fats include oils from olives, coconuts, nuts and seeds (ideally cold pressed, because heavy processing damages fats), as well as green leafy vegetables. Animal products also contain healthy fats. Oily fish is a good source of the omega-3 fats.

We recommend both unsaturated and saturated fats, although saturated fats found in meat and high-fat dairy products should play less of a role in the diet than the unsaturated fats found in vegetables, nuts, seeds and oily fish. As omega-3 is often deficient in the average Western diet, aim to eat omega-3-rich foods daily: flaxseed (also called linseed), walnuts, hempseeds and their oils, oily fish, meat from grass-fed animals and free-range eggs.

Oils can become damaged when heated at high temperatures, and should only be heated to a minimal extent. Saturated fats (such as coconut and animal fats) and monounsaturated fats (such as olive oil) are more stable when heated.

Although butter is a saturated fat, it is far less processed than any type of margarine or low-fat spread and, in moderation, can play a part in a healthy diet.

HERBS AND SPICES Natural flavorings in the form of herbs and spices are a rich source of phytonutrients with powerful health-enhancing properties, including antioxidants and anti-inflammatory capabilities.

We recommend using a variety of herbs and spices on a daily basis. Examples include garlic, ginger, chili, turmeric, rosemary, mint and thyme. Use fresh or dry in salads, cooked dishes and as teas.

Foods to eat in moderate amounts

RED MEAT Important nutrients, including B vitamins and minerals (especially iron), are found in red meat. There is evidence too much red meat can increase the risk of certain cancers, but there is no health risk associated with eating a moderate amount of unprocessed red meat.

We recommend only eating small portions of red meat—approximately the amount that will fit into the palm of your hand. Choose organic or grass-fed meat, if you can, as the nutrient quality is much higher.

DAIRY PRODUCTS Containing a range of vitamins and minerals, dairy products are a good source of protein and healthy fats. Nevertheless, some researchers have questioned whether they are suitable for people with cancer, especially hormone-sensitive cancers. The research shows dairy to be a risk factor in prostate cancer, although there has been little research examining the effects of dairy produce on the health of cancer survivors. Some people find, after anticancer treatment, dairy foods upset their digestion.

We recommend, for people with prostate cancer and those who find milk products difficult to digest, that you keep the amount of dairy products you eat to a minimum. For others, organic and whole-milk yogurt and butter can be used, with minimal amounts of milk and cheese. You might find goat or sheep products are easier to digest.

SOY PRODUCTS   Foods made with soybeans are an important part of traditional Asian diets, such as in the form of tofu, miso or tempeh, but they are a relatively new addition to the Western diet. Like some other plant foods, they contain phytoestrogens; however, soy also contains less-favorable compounds, often termed "antinutrients," that can interfere with nutrient absorption.

We recommend if you eat soy, choose organic types, such as tofu, miso, tempeh and natto, which tend to have lower levels of these antinutrients.

Foods to eat in minimal amounts

These foods have little or no health benefits and are best eaten rarely or avoided.

REFINED GRAINS AND SUGARS   Products made with refined grains, such as white flour and white rice, lose a lot of their nutritional value, including fiber, in the refining process. Eating these refined carbohydrates leads to a rapid rise in blood sugar and encourages unhealthy changes in your body.

We recommend avoiding refined grains and sugary foods as much as possible. Vegetables and fresh or dried fruit are full of natural sweetness and can be used to make healthy puddings, cakes and cookies.

UNHEALTHY/DAMAGED FATS   Fats that have been damaged due to heavy processing are particularly bad for you. Trans-fats are an example. These are mainly found in partially hydrogenated vegetable oils, which are used in commercial potato chips, mayonnaise, cakes, cookies, pastries and deep-fried foods.

We recommend avoiding processed, fatty foods. Instead, prepare cakes, cookies and pastry products at home using butter or oils, such as olive and coconut. Don't heat oils to high temperatures during cooking, as this can cause oxidation and damage the fats, although coconut and canola oils are more stable at higher temperatures.

PROCESSED MEATS   There is evidence to suggest a high intake of processed meats increases the risk of developing some cancers. Processed meats include heavily processed burgers and sausages, salami, bacon and other smoked or cured meats.

We recommend minimizing the amount of processed meat you eat. If you have it occasionally, choose organic products when possible.

BARBECUED, BROILED AND GRIDDLED FOODS   There is evidence that eating lots of barbecued, broiled or griddled foods might increase the risk of certain cancers; however, there is no harm in having any of these occasionally.

We recommend when you cook foods in these ways, particularly meat, don't let them come into direct contact with a naked flame and try not to let them overbrown or burn.

Salt

If processed food forms a large part of your diet, you will most likely be eating too much salt, which can upset the delicate balance of minerals in the body. Whole foods and fresh, unprocessed foods are naturally low in salt. You can use a little good-quality kosher or sea salt in cooking to enhance flavor. Also use herbs, spices, garlic, onions, dried mushrooms, dried tomatoes and lemon juice to further enhance flavor. Seaweed can also add flavor and is a valuable source of iodine, which is often deficient in the modern diet.

Water

Drinking enough water to stay well hydrated is an important part of your healthy-eating plan. The best way to do this is to drink regularly throughout the day. An average adult needs between 1½ quarts and 2 quarts of fluid every day. If you are very physically active or the weather is hot, you might want more. Water, herbal teas and fresh vegetable juices all count toward your fluid intake, but keep fruit juices, sugary drinks, caffeinated drinks and alcohol to a minimum.

Moving forward

Dietary needs can change with time as your health, lifestyle and moods alter. Some foods might be particularly appealing at one time, but less appealing at another. Using the recipes and information in this book you can choose healthy options you can be sure will satisfy you, give you pleasure and support your body.

FOODS TO EAT REGULARLY, ON A DAILY BASIS	FOODS TO EAT IN MODERATE AMOUNTS	FOODS TO EAT IN MINIMAL AMOUNTS
Vegetables and fruit	Red meat	Refined grains and sugars
Protein foods	Dairy products	Unhealthy/damaged fats
Legumes	Soy products	Processed meats/foods
Whole grains		Overbrown, burned and barbecued foods
Healthy fats		Salt
Herbs and spices		
DRINKS		
Water	Coffee	Alcohol

The Power of Food—Where to Find the Nutrients You Need

Many of the natural compounds in whole foods have been shown to discourage cancer growth. Combining them in a meal helps to increase their beneficial properties.

Whether you are undergoing cancer treatment, you are in recovery or wanting to prevent the onset or recurrence of cancer, eating nutrient-rich food is a crucial part of your program. The following charts give examples of nutrient-rich foods, the compounds within them and some possible health benefits.

FOODS	SOME OF THE NATURAL COMPOUNDS	POSSIBLE BENEFITS
Allium vegetables: chives, garlic, leeks, onions, scallions	Allicin, alliin and the enzyme allinase. Diallyl sulfide and S-allyl cysteine. The flavonoid quercetin	Might restrict the growth of cancer cells/tumors and be protective against stomach, gastric and colon cancers. Might inhibit breast, liver and colon cancers. Might help reduce the side effects of radiotherapy. Potent antioxidant and antimicrobial. Quercetin is an antioxidant and might protect against hormone cancers. Immune supportive properties
Citrus fruit: grapefruit lemons, limes, oranges; and celery	Bioflavonoids, such as ellagic acid, hesperidin, rutin. Limonoids, vitamin C	Antioxidant and anti-inflammatory. They support the immune system and inhibit tumor growth

FOODS	SOME OF THE NATURAL COMPOUNDS	POSSIBLE BENEFITS
Cruciferous and green vegetables: broccoli, Brussels sprouts, cabbage, cauliflower, horseradish, kale, mustard greens, radish, spinach, wasabi, watercress	Carotenoids, indole-3-carbinol, sulforophane, vitamins C, E and K	Disrupt tumor formation and growth. Promote cancer cell death. Antioxidant and anti-inflammatory
Mushrooms: button, cordyceps, enoki, maitake, reishi, shiitake	Lentinan, polysaccharides	Shiitake mushrooms contain 1:3 beta-glucan polysaccharides that support immunity and destroy cancer cells. Maitake, cordyceps and reishi encourage the immune system to identify and destroy cancer cells
Orange/yellow vegetables and fruit: apricots, bell peppers, carrots, mangoes, pumpkins, squash, sweet potatoes, watermelon	Carotenoids, particularly beta-carotene, lutein, lycopene	An immune-enhancing effect. They have been shown to inhibit cancer cell formation and are potent antioxidants. Some studies have shown beta-carotene supplements can reduce cancer risk by 40 percent. (Smokers, however, should not supplement with synthetic beta-carotene.)
Red vegetables and fruit: acai berries, beets, blueberries, cherries, cranberries, eggplants, figs, grapes, pomegranates, raspberries, red cabbage, red plums, strawberries	Anthocyanins, ellagic acid, flavonoids, oligomeric proanthocyanidins, resveratrol	Protect against DNA damage. Reduce the rate of cancer cell growth and cause cancer cell death. They have antiestrogen activity, are anti-inflammatory and support immune activity. Many of these compounds have been shown to prevent breast and prostate cancers

FOODS	SOME OF THE NATURAL COMPOUNDS	POSSIBLE BENEFITS
Tomatoes	Carotenoids, lycopene, vitamin C	Inhibit tumor formation and carcinogenic activity. Harvard Medical School found eating 10 servings a week could reduce prostate cancer risk by 40 percent. Fat helps the absorption of lycopene
Beans and legumes	Fiber, isoflavones, phytoestrogens	Inhibit tumor formation. Might protect against certain hormonal cancers, such as breast and prostate. Reduce the risk of atherosclerosis, heart disease and osteoporosis
Oily fish: anchovies, mackerel, pilchards, salmon, sardines, trout	Omega-3 fats, vitamin D	Anticarcinogenic and anti-inflammatory. Regulates the immune system. Slows the growth of tumors and prevents their spread. Effective against hormone-dependent cancers. Avoid eating larger fish, such as shark, swordfish, marlin and tuna
Soy	Genistein, isoflavones, excellent source of complete protein to replace meat	Tissue repair. Can help to balance hormones. Ideally use the whole-food product to supply isoflavones rather than an isolated supplement. Choose organic, non-GM soy, preferably fermented
Variety meat, especially kidneys and liver	B vitamins, iron, selenium, vitamin D	Increases energy and circulation of oxygen. Antioxidant. Selenium might protect against certain cancers, such as breast and prostate cancer

FOODS	SOME OF THE NATURAL COMPOUNDS	POSSIBLE BENEFITS
Apple cider vinegar	Malic acid, pectin, potassium	Supports digestive health and secretion of digestive enzymes. Lowers glycemic index/load of meals
Butter, ghee	Butyric acid, conjugated linoleic acid (CLA), vitamins A and D	Improve intestinal health. CLA is shown to suppress cancer cells
Coconut: flesh, oil, water and milk	Caprylic acid, lauric acid, medium chain triglycerides	Antimicrobial and anticancer properties. Easy to digest
Fermented foods, such as live yogurt, miso, sauerkraut	Healthy bacteria (probiotics)	Support digestion, immune function and intestinal health
Flaxseed (linseed) and its oil, nuts, seeds, whole grains	Lignans, magnesium, phytosterols	Modulate estrogen activity and enhance immune function. Antioxidant activity, antibacterial, antiviral and antifungal
Olive oil and avocado oil	Oleic acid, omega-9 fatty acids	Support blood sugar levels. Antioxidant, free-radical scavenger
Sea vegetables: arame, dulse, kelp, kombu, wakame	Fucoidan, iodine	Fucoidans are starchlike (polysaccharide) molecules with anti-inflammatory and antiviral properties. They are immune enhancing and might reduce the risk of breast cancer. Iodine assists thyroid function and improves metabolism
Tea (matcha, white, green, black), dark chocolate	Polyphenols, such as catechins, including epigallocatechin gallate (EGCG)	Antioxidant, anti-inflammatory and antiangiogenic. Modulate hormone activity and support immune function

HERBS AND SPICES	SOME OF THE NATURAL COMPOUNDS	POSSIBLE BENEFITS
Basil, mint, oregano, rosemary, thyme	Essential oils of the tarpene family	Reduce the spread of cancer cells by blocking enzymes needed to invade other tissue
Cilantro/coriander	Leaves, essential oils in seeds	A digestive aid. Anti-inflammatory and antimicrobial
Fennel	Coumarin compounds, such as anethole	Reduces inflammation by influencing cell signaling
Parsley	Carotenes, chlorophyll, folic acid, iron, vitamin C	Inhibits the cancer-causing properties of fried foods. A nerve stimulant, useful in energy drinks
Peppermint	Perillyl alcohol, also contains rosmarinic acid	Inhibits the growth of tumors and is a powerful antioxidant
Sage	Flavonoids, rosmarinic acid	Has blood-sugar lowering effects. Antimicrobial and antifungal
Chilies	Capsaicin	Antimicrobial. Might be particularly effective against certain types of skin cancer
Cinnamon	Essential oils from the bark, such as cinnamyl acetate	Helps to balance blood sugar, helps insomnia and optimizes circulation
Cloves	Beta-caryophyllene, eugenol	Might prevent digestive-tract cancers. Offers protection from environmental pollution. Used in the treatment of joint inflammation. A mild anesthetic

HERBS AND SPICES	SOME OF THE NATURAL COMPOUNDS	POSSIBLE BENEFITS
Ginger	Gingerols	Anti-inflammatory, stimulates digestion and soothes the intestinal tract. Promotes circulation
Saffron	Carotenoids, dimethylcrocetin, safranal	Immune-boosting anticarcinogenic, antioxidant and antidepressant
Turmeric	Curcumin is the main active ingredient in this curry spice	Antioxidant activity and anti-inflammatory, stimulates cancer cell death (apoptosis)

This is just a selection of whole foods and their benefits, and it shows how many contain natural health-giving properties. Don't feel it is essential to eat specific foods because of their healthy properties, if they don't appeal to you. Always be guided by your taste, and include your favorite foods as well as the ones above that you prefer. Just as we adopt a whole-person approach to our well-being, we should also adopt a synergistic approach to food and meals by combining different foods in one meal or a snack.

When planning meals, eat a variety of whole foods in combination, and avoid concentrating on one particular food or compound because of its specific benefit. Choose a food rather than a supplement; enjoy a curry flavored with turmeric and made with meat, poultry or a vegetarian protein, plus vegetables, rather than taking a turmeric supplement. You will benefit from the anti-inflammatory properties of the curcumin as well as the anti-inflammatory and antioxidant benefits from the healthy fats you cook with, the other curry spices and the foods you have included.

Managing Treatment & Side Effects

What you eat during your cancer treatment really matters, because it helps to keep you strong and can also help you deal with any problems caused by the treatment. This chapter looks at some of the side effects you can expect from treatment and explains what and how to eat to help you feel better.

Our healthy-eating approach can form the basis of anything you do before, during and after treatment; however, there can be times when you need to adapt our guidelines. Your body, your illness and your circumstances are unique, so use this information accordingly. You might also want to talk to a specialist to receive personalized advice.

Fatigue

Feeling tired is the most common symptom people with cancer experience during and after treatment. Use food to obtain the energy and nutrients that you need.

• Be prepared. Do your shopping online. Cook when you are not tired. Make larger quantities of food than you need for one meal and freeze some of it for other days.

• Have nutritious, homemade soups, because they are easy to digest and do not contain energy-depleting additives present in commercial foods.

• Drink plenty of fluids, because dehydration depletes energy. Try the juices described in this book. Have a chocolate drink, using your choice of milk or milk substitute. Dark chocolate has a remarkable effect on energy levels. It can also lift your mood.

• Have healthy, nutritious snacks: fresh fruit with nuts or seeds, dried fruit (figs, dates and apricots), dark chocolate, boiled eggs, yogurt, chicken liver or sardine pâté. Your body is able to digest snacks and small meals better than one large meal.

• Aim to be a healthy weight.

Loss of appetite and nausea

A loss of appetite is a complex symptom. It can be caused by treatment or by the cancer itself. Changes to your sense of taste and smell, experiencing a dry mouth, nausea, diarrhea, constipation, slower digestion of your food, fatigue, low mood or depression, anxiety, pain, breathlessness and infection might all cause you to lose your appetite. Ask for help from your medical team to address what can be treated.

• Try different foods and find what you enjoy most. Sometimes eating smaller meals more frequently can help.

• Always go for the healthier choices. Avoid foods that are difficult to digest, such as deep-fried foods.

• Sometimes gentle foods, such as oatmeal, are the easiest to eat when you are not hungry or you feel sick. Oatmeal is quick and easy to make and has calories to sustain you, as well as antioxidants and fiber. Add some ground seeds and nuts, banana, honey, cinnamon and berries, poached fruit or plums.

• Avoid strong smells, because these can trigger nausea. When you are nauseous, drink plenty of water, mild vegetable juices and herb teas, such as peppermint, which can aid digestion and, therefore, avoids the side effect of nausea. Ginger can also help reduce your sickness, so use it in teas and food.

• To improve your appetite, have a walk in the fresh air before you eat.

Changes in taste and smell

Some chemotherapy drugs, as well as certain antibiotics, painkillers and steroids, can make food taste salty, bitter or metallic. Radiotherapy to the head and neck region can damage the taste buds and alter your sense of smell or change taste.

• Avoid red meats, which can have a particularly metallic taste.

• Flavor foods with herbs, spices and lemon juice.

• You might find cold foods more appealing than hot foods.

Difficulty swallowing, oral thrush and mouth ulcers

Swallowing problems and mouth ulcers can be a result of chemotherapy or radiation to the neck or chest area. You might be susceptible to infections, such as oral thrush, which can make swallowing painful, because the cancer and/or its treatment suppresses your immune system.

- If possible, consume fresh vegetable juices to boost your nutrient intake. Cabbage juice is soothing to the throat and the rest of the digestive tract. Mix it with other vegetables and fruit to enhance the flavor.
- Consume softer healthy foods, such as bananas, mashed root vegetables (carrot, parsnip, rutabaga, sweet potato), rice pudding, homemade soups and casseroles and cooked fruit. Braise tougher foods like meat, to tenderize them, and mix them with softer foods to make them easier to eat. You can try blending them in a blender or food processor, if necessary.
- Take a sip of water (or vegetable juice) between each bite of food, so the liquid helps wash the food down between mouthfuls.
- Use a straw if necessary for liquids and blended foods.
- Avoid salty, spicy or acidic foods to prevent extra irritation to your mouth.
- Consume as many immune-supporting foods as possible, particularly vegetables and fruit, onions and garlic, shiitake mushrooms, herbs and spices.

Digestive problems: bloating and flatulence, or slower digestion of food

Cancer, its treatment and even dietary changes, such as rapidly switching to a raw or whole-food diet, can all cause digestive problems. Some people who have had surgery, radiotherapy and/or certain types of chemotherapy become unable to digest fats, carbohydrates (such as lactose found in dairy products) and proteins (such as the gluten found in wheat and other grains). This can be temporary or permanent. When it happens, it causes abdominal cramps, bloating and flatulence. If raw foods or legumes are new to your diet, introduce them gradually.

It is important to discuss any concerns with a professional, such as a doctor or nutritionally trained health-care provider.

Diarrhea

Treatment, or the cancer itself, can cause diarrhea, and it can also be the result of stress, food intolerances or a viral or bacterial infection. If the diarrhea is severe and longer than two days, seek help from your doctor.

• Drink plenty of fluids to replace those lost.

• Avoid all dairy products, because the lactose in milk can make diarrhea worse.

• Avoid hot or very cold drinks.

• Avoid caffeine.

• Avoid greasy and/or heavily spiced foods.

• You might need to reduce your intake of high-fiber foods, but only until the diarrhea improves. In this case, avoid legumes, whole grains (use white flour, pasta and rice in the short term instead) and raw vegetables and fruit (try peeled, cooked vegetables and fruit instead).

• The insoluble fiber and pectin in apples helps bowel regularity, and might relieve both constipation and diarrhea.

Constipation

Like diarrhea, constipation can be due to the cancer itself or its treatment. It can also be caused by poor diet lacking in sufficient fiber, low fluid intake and/or decreased physical activity and weakness.

• Drink plenty of fluids; warm drinks, such as herb teas can be particularly helpful.

• Eat more high-fiber foods, such as whole grains, vegetables and fruit (especially oranges and apples).

• Eat dried fruit, especially prunes and figs, to help keep the bowels moving.

• Gentle exercise might be beneficial.

• Massaging the tummy gently can help to ease blockages.

• Eat slowly and chew well to help digestion.

Maintaining a Healthy Weight

Until recently, people were advised to eat whatever they wanted during cancer treatment to avoid losing weight. Modern knowledge challenges this and stresses the importance of eating a balanced, nutritious diet to maintain a healthy weight.

Weight gain

When you have cancer, you can put on excessive weight for a number of reasons:

- You have certain types of cancer, such as breast, prostate, endometrial, ovarian, colorectal and brain cancer, in which hormonal changes and treatment can encourage weight gain.
- You are taking certain medications, such as steroids and hormonal treatments. Contrary to expectation, many people can also put on excess weight during chemotherapy, as well as other treatments.
- You are feeling tired or stressed. You can then turn to eating comfort foods.
- You don't do enough physical activity because of fatigue, discomfort, low mood or habit, or for other reasons.
- You find it difficult to change unhealthy eating habits, especially at times of crisis.

To help you achieve a healthy weight, follow the principles set out in this book. Research has shown that a plant-based diet can encourage weight loss in those who are overweight, particularly if combined with regular physical activity.

Maintain a reasonable level of physical activity, without overdoing it. Physical activity, such as walking, will help you to deal with fatigue, as well as burning calories and lifting your mood. When exercising aim to lift your spirits as well as increasing your energy. Use meditation, visualization or relaxation to support yourself and maintain your resolve.

Another useful way to help avoid weight gain is to eat mindfully. Research shows when we eat slowly and chew well, we feel full quicker and, therefore, eat less. Remember, however, each one of us is different. How we deal with weight gain will depend on our circumstances, and these can also change and influence our resolve to do what is best for us. Small changes in eating patterns can make a big difference after a while. If you have a setback it is always worth trying again.

Weight loss

People with cancer can lose weight for many reasons: as a direct effect of the tumor or following cancer treatment (surgery, chemotherapy, radiotherapy). Cancer is a complicated disease and the disease processes it uses for its survival can sometimes lead to weight loss, often accompanied by a loss of appetite. In certain types of cancer, including lung and pancreatic cancer, this is more common.

If you are losing weight, you might need to eat extra calories, proteins, healthy fats and other nutrients. Healthy, calorie-rich foods include nuts and seeds, dried fruit (figs, dates and prunes), oily fish, avocados, dark chocolate, nut and seed butters, coconut milk and whole-milk yogurt. Try our Blueberry Avocado Build-Up Shake, for example. Don't be tempted to fill yourself up with unhealthy fats or sugar.

It might also help you if you follow an anti-inflammatory diet and lifestyle to reduce inflammation, which is linked to cancer growth:

- Eat foods that have anti-inflammatory properties (fruit and vegetables, whole grains, legumes, fish, olive oil and herbs)—see The Power of Food, page 24.
- Avoid foods that lead to inflammation (oils high in omega-6 fatty acids, foods containing trans-fats, commercially fried foods)—see page 12.
- As well as eating healthily, do regular exercise, because it inhibits the production of compounds, such as some prostaglandins, which contribute to inflammation.
- Have some exposure to sunshine to create adequate vitamin D: 15 minutes a day without sunscreen, but avoid burning. Adequate vitamin D is essential for immune system functioning and is very commonly deficient in cancer patients.
- Consider taking omega-3 supplements. A diet rich in omega-3 fatty acids has been shown to help people with weight loss in the advanced stages of cancer.

How to Eat Well

It takes just a moment to make the decision to improve your diet, but making those improvements actually happen is a daily process—albeit an exciting one—of discovering new foods, new recipes and new eating routines. This section offers some practical hints and tips on how to make those changes.

Moving on, step by step

• Too many changes at once can be overwhelming and stressful, both physically and emotionally. Do things at a gradual pace that suits you. Even small changes can bring positive benefits that will help to keep you motivated.

• Take time to restock your cupboards and refrigerator with whole foods.

• Get support. If you have friends or family offering to help, ask them to prepare a meal for you, perhaps something you can freeze to eat at a later date. Many of the recipes in this book can be frozen or will keep for a few days in the refrigerator.

• Get advice. Talk to people who are familiar with healthy cooking and ask them for their tips, tricks and ideas.

• Buy standby foods for off-days. A selection of healthy frozen foods is a useful option for days when cooking requires too much effort. Canned products, such as legumes, tomatoes and fish, and nut and seed butters, are also handy to have readily available, but choose those without added sugar or salt. If you always have nuts and fruit at home, you can easily prepare a smoothie.

• Grow your own. Consider growing some herbs in pots, or even planting a small vegetable plot. Freshly picked food, direct from your garden, will be bursting with goodness. Plus, there's the satisfaction of producing vegetables yourself, and the increased endorphins and physical activity will help your well-being.

• Expect more changes. Make healthy eating a habit, but accept that your tastes might change as your treatment, health and activity levels progress, so don't feel bound to one particular choice of diet.

Enjoy your food

Good food does more than provide nutrition. A tasty meal, particularly when shared with others, is enjoyable, making it good for the body and for the soul. Sometimes new routines can enhance that enjoyment.

• Relish your food. Take time to eat, savor and digest your meal.

• Show love and respect for food, life and self.

• Be aware of your environment when you eat. Try to make your surroundings pleasant, comfortable and relaxing.

• When you do allow yourself a treat, feel good about it; for example, focus on the beneficial aspects of the food, such as the antioxidants in coffee, red wine or chocolate, and know that the occasional treat can boost your endorphin levels, helping you to feel good.

The connection between food and mood

The food we eat alters the chemical balance of our bodies and affects our physical, emotional and spiritual health. Large and rapid ups and downs in the levels of blood glucose (sugar) are linked to changes in mood and energy. After a sugary snack, blood glucose can spike and then very quickly drop again to a relatively low level. This can lead to irritability, light-headedness, lower concentration and tiredness, as in the "post-lunch dip." To help stabilize blood sugar levels, try some of the following:

• Eat regular meals. If you feel hungry, have a snack midmorning and/or afternoon.

• Combine protein, fat and fiber at each meal and snack. Eating low-GL meals (see page 13) helps to regulate the release of glucose and moderates mood. A protein-rich breakfast will help to reduce cravings later in the day.

• Drink plenty of fluids between meals. Brain function requires a large percentage of the body's intake of fluids, so have a glass of water near you to avoid dehydration. Avoid sugary drinks, sodas, fruit juices and too much tea or coffee.

• Include plenty of omega-3-rich foods to maintain a healthy brain, which is largely comprised of these fats. Omega-3 can also help to control insulin function.

Digestion and stress

Have you ever eaten a meal but barely tasted it? Or maybe had a snack without even registering it? Hasty, distracted eating when you are busy or stressed makes it difficult for your body to digest even the healthiest food.

How to improve your digestion

• Reduce stress when eating. A calming routine at mealtimes helps you to switch from your daily worries to the pleasure of eating. Take a little time (5 to 10 minutes) to sit down and stimulate your appetite to begin the digestive process. Try relaxation or imagery, or simply take two deep breaths before you eat. You might want to light a candle or put a vase of flowers on the table.

• Savor your food. Notice its color and freshness, smell your food and enjoy its aroma, use as many of your senses as you can, even before you begin to eat. Taking time to anticipate meals prepares the digestive system.

• Eat slowly and mindfully. Chew every mouthful thoroughly, focusing on the nutrients, energy and pleasure your meal is giving you. This will stimulate your body to produce more enzymes and make digestion more efficient. If you are in the habit of eating quickly, try putting your knife and fork down between mouthfuls.

• Take a break. Let your digestive system rest between meals. Constant snacking is only necessary and useful if you have very poor blood sugar balance.

• Don't drink too much while eating, as this might dilute your digestive juices.

• Avoid eating late at night. This can raise insulin levels, increasing belly fat and puts additional pressure on the digestive system as you try to sleep.

• Cook your food, if you are having digestion problems. Cooking food can help to break down some of the fibrous and tough material in the outer plant or animal membranes. Raw food, although nutritious and flavorsome, can be difficult to manage on occasions if your digestive system is affected by illness, treatments or drugs. Raw juices, however, do not contain fiber, but are an easier way to get essential, concentrated nutrients than eating raw vegetables.

• Spice it up. Use spices or herbs with most meals (page 20). Eating sour and/or bitter foods can help with any symptoms of indigestion you might have.

Natural condiments from the pantry

There are lots of natural ingredients you can add to dishes to create food bursting with flavors, and many of them possess powerful health-enhancing properties.

DEPTH AND RICHNESS	QUALITIES, BENEFITS	USE
Barley miso	Fermented soy and barley. Rich in phytoestrogens	Can be used for pungent salad dressings or in savory dishes, such as lentils or beans
Unsweetened cacao powder, nibs or cocoa	A naturally rich source of antioxidants and magnesium	Add 1 tbsp. to chili or lasagne. Adds depth to smoothies and sweet dishes
Sweet/white miso	Fermented soy and rice. Light in color, texture and flavor. Rich in phytoestrogens	Suitable for salads and stir-fries. Delicious in marinades and soups
Tahini	A sesame paste rich in calcium, zinc and essential omega-6 fatty acids	Adds a nutty texture and flavor to dips, stir-fries, salads and dressings, or use as a spread on crackers

SAVORY AND SALTY	QUALITIES, BENEFITS	USE
Anchovies	Can be used from a jar or can. Add saltiness and bring out the flavor of other ingredients	Use as a whole garnish for salads or grain dishes. Can be crushed into stir-fries and soups
Capers	Easy to source, available in jars. Rich in health-promoting flavonoids, such as rutin and quercetin	Add a pungent and sour taste to dishes containing fish and grains
Nori/seaweed flakes	Rich in minerals and easy to use. Adds a slight saltiness to dishes. Good source of iodine	Can enhance the flavors of other ingredients. Great in soups, stews and added to salads
Nutritional yeast flakes	Inert yeast flakes in a carton. Rich in B vitamins. Give a yeasty/cheese flavor	Flavor balances well with nutmeg. Add to sauces and dressings. Great for flavoring vegan dishes
Pesto	Rich in flavor. Antioxidant benefits from its herb base	Add to stir-fries, pasta, potatoes, salad dressings and eggs
Tamari/shoyu	Good-quality, naturally fermented soy sauces. Tamari is gluten-free	To add saltiness and depth. Use sparingly, because high in salt
Umeboshi vinegar/ume seasoning	An alkalizing fermented plum vinegar. Useful as a digestive aid	Add to stews, salads, stir-fries. Can be used in marinades
Wine/apple cider vinegar	Helps digestion and to stabilize blood glucose levels by reducing the glycemic index/load	Choose a good-quality, naturally fermented vinegar. Add to salads, stews and stir-fries
Yeast extract	Rich in B vitamins (use in small amounts)	Adds pungency and saltiness to soups, casseroles and stir-fries

Although sugar should be as scant as possible in the diet, these healthier sweeteners have a lower glycemic index than sugar, but it is still important to use them sparingly.

SWEETNESS	QUALITIES	USE
Apple juice concentrate (AJC)	Adds depth and balance to sweet and savory dishes. High in fructose, so use sparingly	Useful for balancing the flavor of seaweed. Excellent in salads. Adds sweetness to a cake batter
Lucuma	A nutrient-dense fruit from Peru, tasting like butterscotch	Use in ice creams and smoothies
Maca	A nutritious Peruvian root vegetable with a naturally sweet, caramel flavor. Used to modulate the effects of stress and to support hormonal health	Delicious added to drinks, cakes and desserts. Commonly found in powdered form
Molasses	A bitter edge to an overall sweetness. Can be very dominant in taste. A high mineral content, including iron, calcium and magnesium	Use for sweet and savory dishes. A little goes a long way
Stevia	A naturally sweet plant with a low glycemic index	A little goes a long way. Supplied as granules
Xylitol	A natural sugar primarily derived from birch trees with minimal impact on blood sugar levels	Can be used like superfine sugar, in cakes, puddings and other desserts

Frequently Asked Questions

Why is organic food so important?

For some people, organic food is preferred for its better taste, or because of their concern for the environment; for others, it's their disquiet about the "cocktail" effect of multiple residues on human health. Safety standards exist for pesticide use in agriculture; however, where one additive might be safe in small amounts, this doesn't necessarily mean that in combination with others it is also safe. Organic foods are produced without the use of synthetic pesticides and chemical fertilizers. They do not contain genetically modified organisms and are not processed using irradiation, industrial solvents or chemical food additives.

A number of studies have indicated there is a benefit to eating organic rather than industrially grown food in terms of safety (pesticide or chemical contamination and use of antibiotics), nutritional value, taste and environmental impact. It is, however, vital you eat a variety of foods, rather than restricting your diet because you choose not to eat foods unless they are organically grown.

Wash all fruit and vegetables thoroughly with water. If using conventionally grown fruit and vegetables, adding a little vinegar or lemon juice to the washing water can help to remove surface chemicals, as will peeling.

If I don't eat dairy, what is the healthiest way to eat for strong bones?

Research is very clear on this: those who eat plenty of fruit and vegetables daily have healthy bones. This is due to the alkalizing effect of fruit and vegetables, as well as due to the vitamin K, phytoestrogens and other bioactive nutrients found in abundance in these foods. Add to your diet small fish with bones, such as canned sardines, as well as eating legumes, nuts and seeds (particularly sesame seeds and tahini), leafy green vegetables (such as cabbage, kale, spinach, parsley and watercress) and whole grains, all of which are rich in calcium. You get from these foods all the goodness that you need for your bones. Other dairy alternatives include:

- Oat, soy, rice and nut milks. Oat is particularly recommended, because it is easy to digest and usually free from added sugars.
- Healthy oils, such as olive oil or coconut oil, to spread or drizzle over bread.
- Alternatives to cheese include dips, pâtés and nut or seed butters.
- Soy yogurts are available; choose the unsweetened variety.
- Oat and nut creams are available.

Why should I reduce my coffee intake when it makes me feel so alert?

Caffeine is found in certain drinks, such as tea (the black, green and white varieties), and especially coffee. It is also found in some foods, such as chocolate. Caffeine can increase the body's production of stress hormones, including epinephrine (also known as adrenaline), hence the feel-good factor. Increased epinephrine puts additional stress on the body's reserves of nutrients, however, and this process can also raise blood glucose levels. For this reason coffee is not recommended in large quantities or to be drunk regularly. It is particularly important to minimize caffeine intake during times of stress. If you do drink coffee, do so in moderation and enjoy it.

Can I drink alcohol?

Some alcoholic drinks, such as red wine, contain compounds with beneficial antioxidant properties, such as resveratrol. These properties are enhanced if organic products are used; however, alcohol itself offers very little benefit to the body, apart from its relaxation effects, and can place stress on the liver as well as undermining general health. Research evidence clearly shows alcohol can increase the risk of certain cancers, as well as heart disease and high blood pressure.

If you choose to drink alcohol, ideally keep it for special occasions and celebrations, and enjoy it in moderation. Those drinking alcohol more regularly should not exceed two drinks a week. Antioxidant compounds similar to those in red wine can be obtained by eating a diet rich in fresh vegetables and fruit.

Is it a good idea to become vegetarian or vegan?

Every individual has a different requirement for nutrients, and while some people thrive eating animal products, others don't, or choose to avoid them. We encourage people to eat a plant-based diet and avoid processed meat, but we do not recommend avoiding animal products completely, because they can contribute valuable, easily utilized protein and iron, as well as other nutrients to the diet, including omega-3 fats (if the animals are grass fed and organic/free range), selenium, vitamins A and B12 and other B vitamins. If meat is particularly hard to digest, or undesirable, eating small amounts of dairy—milk, yogurt and butter—and moderate amounts of eggs and fish is advisable. If you choose to avoid animal products:

• Avoid restricting your food choices to just one or two foods to replace the protein and other nutrients present in animal products. A wide variety and combination of foods is essential, particularly if you are avoiding animal products. Seeds, nuts and legumes are all good sources of protein.

• Eat a variety of nutrient-rich plant foods to provide sufficient amino acids (the protein building blocks), vitamins, minerals and essential fatty acids. Plant sources with good profiles include: quinoa, buckwheat, amaranth, hempseed and soy.

• Eat seaweeds, which contain vitamins, minerals, amino acids and iodine.

• Certain plant foods—legumes (peas and beans), whole grains and seeds—contain oxalate and phytate, which inhibit calcium absorption. Sprouting significantly reduces the phytate content, so using a combination of sprouted seeds and grains is beneficial. Phytates can also restrict iron absorption from plant foods (iron-rich foods include legumes, seeds and nuts). The inhibiting effect can be lessened by including vitamin C-rich foods in your diet.

Is it safe to eat soy?

Soybeans are a source of fiber, vitamins and minerals, as well as phytoestrogens. Phytoestrogens, when obtained from a variety of plant foods and as part of a balanced diet, can have positive benefits for the body, such as regulating certain hormones. Other sources of phytoestrogens include certain legumes, seeds, grains and vegetables. Phytoestrogens in food, rather than from supplements, don't seem to be a risk factor for cancer, so they do not need to be avoided. For vegetarians, soy products can provide a valuable source of complete protein. We do not, however, recommend the use of soy foods in large amounts (more than four servings weekly), because of the antinutrient factors (see page 21). Also, raw or sprouted soybeans might interfere with thyroid gland activity and should not be eaten by those with already compromised thyroid health. Cooked soybeans do not have the same effect.

Should I take supplements?

It is always best, if you can, to eat whole foods rather than taking supplements. The multiple bioactive components in food work together (synergistically), so the combined effect is greater than the effect of the individual components.

However, alongside a healthy diet, and particularly if you are not able to eat sufficient quantities of food, you might wish to add a little extra nutritional support. If this is your choice:

• Always keep to recommended dosage instructions and take products designed for general nutritional support unless under professional guidance.

• Always inform your medical team of the supplements you are taking.

• Because there is still limited research on the use of supplements during treatments, we recommend you stop taking them during chemotherapy and radiotherapy, unless advised otherwise by your medical team.

Seven-Day Menu Plans

The following daily menus can be used as a basis when you plan your meals for the week. Mix and match as you like. You can also choose to minimize cooking by eating leftovers for lunch the next day or by cooking a larger quantity for eating another day.

Nonvegetarian

BREAKFAST	LUNCH	DINNER	SNACK
Mixed Seed Granola, with yogurt (p.56)	Pan-Fried Squid with Red Cabbage & Walnuts (p.83)	Persian Quinoa Omega Bowl (p.117)	Ginger, Almond & Chocolate Cookies (p.141)
Spanish Baked Eggs (p.63)	Warm Lentil & Bean Salad (p.91)	Chicken & Cashew Stir-Fry (p.94)	Coconut Rice Pudding (p.157)
Almond & Pear Oatmeal (p.144)	Garlic & Bean Soup with Pesto (p.71)	Roasted Sea Bass with Olives & Tomatoes (p.103)	Baked Lemon Cheesecake (p.123)
Sardines with Roasted Tomatoes (p.65)	Wilted Kale Salad with Toasted Seeds (p.87)	Venison with Zesty Gremolata (p.101)	Wheatgrass Energizer (p.151)
Flaxseed, Apricot & Cinnamon Muffins (p.59)	Sicilian Shrimp (p.82)	Spaghetti with Lemon & Broccoli (p.114)	Super-Berry Yogurt Sorbet (p.126)
Blueberry & Avocado Build-Up Shake (p.142)	Noodle, Shallot & Shiitake Salad (p.148)	Turkey & Pistachio Korma (p.98)	Matcha & Mango Shake (p.51)
Star Anise-Poached Plums with Ginger-Nut Cream (p.55)	Super-Greens Salad with Chicken (p.77)	Mixed Seafood Pie (p.109)	Italian Crackers & Bean Dip (p.158)

Vegetarian

BREAKFAST	LUNCH	DINNER	SNACK
Mixed Seed Granola (p.56) with soy or coconut yogurt	Hoisin Tempeh Skewers (p.84)	Warm Eggplant, Roots & Chickpea Salad (p.113)	Coconut Rice Pudding (p.157)
Spiced Flatbreads (p.135), with hummus or nut butter	Creamy Cauliflower Soup (p.72)	Hempseed & Nut Burgers (p.116), Celery Root, Apple & Fennel Rémoulade (p.88)	Stamina-Boosting Beet Juice (p.151)
Green Hemp Shake (p.51), Date & Lucuma Cocoa Bar (p.60)	Bell Pepper Bisque with Chili Cream (p.74)	Roasted Tempeh with Pipérade Sauce (p.110)	Matcha Tea & Banana Bread (p.130)
Date & Lucuma Cocoa Bar (p.60)	Garlic & Bean Soup with Pesto (p.71)	Persian Quinoa Omega Bowl (p.117)	Super-Berry Yogurt Sorbet (p.126)
Star Anise-Poached Plums with Ginger-Nut Cream (p.55)	Mixed Sea Vegetable & Cucumber Salad (p.90)	Spaghetti with Lemon & Broccoli (p.114)	Coconut-Cocoa Booster (p.154)
Almond & Pear Oatmeal (p.144)	Super-Greens Salad with Nut Dressing (p.77)	Red Cabbage & Walnuts (p.83), Italian Crackers & Bean Dip (p.158)	Chocolate & Beet Bar (p.133)
Flaxseed, Apricot & Cinnamon Muffins (p.59)	Wilted Kale Salad with Toasted Seeds (p.87)	Warm Lentil & Bean Salad (p.91), Spiced Flatbreads (p.135)	Baked Lemon Cheesecake (p.123)

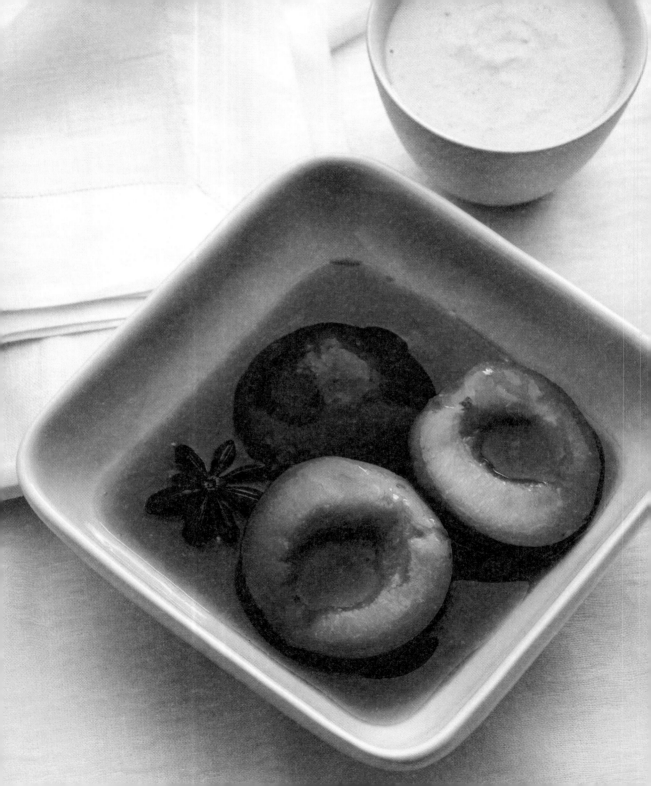

Shakes, Juices, Smoothies & Breakfasts

A shake, juice or smoothie contains beneficial ingredients in a form that is easy to take, making it useful for breakfast or as a snack, particularly if you find your appetite is low or you're just too tired to cook a meal. Other tempting breakfast options in this chapter include Flaxseed, Apricot & Cinnamon Muffins, omega-rich Mixed Seed Granola, warming Star Anise-Poached Plums with Ginger-Nut Cream and speedy Spanish Baked Eggs. Whether it's a quick pick-me-up you need or something to keep you going during treatment, the recipes in this chapter are packed with nutrients to support your body and are designed to reinvigorate your appetite, bolster your energy levels and kick-start your metabolism.

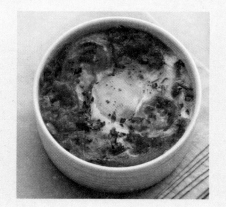

Opposite: Star Anise-Poached Plums with Ginger-Nut Cream (page 55)
Above: Spanish Baked Eggs (page 63)

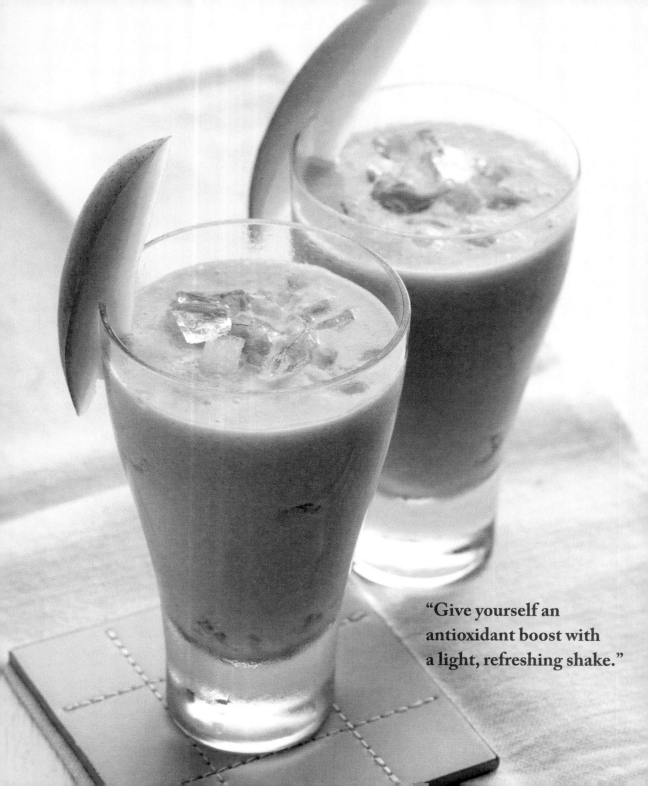

"Give yourself an antioxidant boost with a light, refreshing shake."

◄ Matcha & Mango Shake

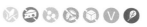

1 Put the almonds in a blender or food processor with 2 cups plus 2 tablespoons water and process until smooth. Strain through a fine strainer, if you prefer.

2 Add the mango and the matcha and process again until thick and creamy. Drink immediately, served with ice and mango, if you like, or store in the refrigerator up to 2 days.

SERVES 2, 1 cup each
PREPARATION TIME 5 minutes

scant ½ cup blanched almonds
1 ripe mango, peeled, seeded and diced
1 teaspoon matcha green tea
ice, to serve
mango slices, to serve (optional)

NUTRITIONAL INFORMATION PER SERVING
Protein 9.4g, **Carbohydrates** 11.8g of which sugars 11.1g,
Fat 16.9g of which saturates 1.4g, **Calories** 234

HEALTH BENEFITS
Matcha is an antioxidant-rich powdered Japanese green tea. The whole leaves are used, making matcha more potent and higher in antioxidants than brewed green tea.

Green Hemp Shake

1 Put all the ingredients into a blender or food processor and process until smooth. Drink immediately or store in the refrigerator up to 1 day.

SERVES 2, 1 cup each
PREPARATION TIME 5 minutes

¼ cup hemp protein powder
  or shelled hempseed
1 ripe mango, peeled, stoned and diced
a pinch cinnamon
1¾ cups coconut water or water
2 large handfuls spinach leaves, cos
  lettuce or kale
a pinch stevia, if needed, to taste

NUTRITIONAL INFORMATION PER SERVING
Protein 10g, **Carbohydrates** 19.9g of which sugars 10.3g,
Fats 2.6g of which saturates 0.1g, **Calories** 142

HEALTH BENEFITS
Hemp protein powder is an easy and healthy way to increase your intake of quality protein and omega-3 and -6 essential fats. It also helps stabilize blood sugar levels.

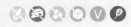

Green Elixir

SERVES 1, 1 cup
PREPARATION TIME 5 minutes

2 celery sticks
½ cucumber
2 large handfuls kale
¾-inch piece fresh gingerroot
1 lemon
2 apples
ice cubes, to serve (optional)
1 tablespoon seeds or nuts, to serve

1 Put all the ingredients through an electric juicer and drink immediately or store in the refrigerator up to 1 day. Serve with ice, if you like, and with 1 tablespoon seeds or nuts.

NUTRITIONAL INFORMATION PER SERVING
Protein 3.6g, **Carbohydrates** 19.9g of which sugars 18.6g, **Fat** 1.2g of which saturates 0.1g, **Calories** 100

HEALTH BENEFITS
This light and cleansing juice contains ginger to ease nausea and digestive upsets. (If you have thyroid problems, limit your intake of brassicas, such as raw kale, as they can have a goitrogenic effect, lowering the function of the thyroid and reducing metabolism.)

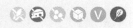

Digestive Healer

SERVES 1, 1 cup
PREPARATION TIME 5 minutes

½ pineapple, peeled (core included)
½-inch piece fresh gingerroot
1 handful parsley
3½ ounces baby spinach leaves
½ cucumber
1 tablespoon aloe vera juice (optional)
1 tablespoon seeds or nuts, to serve

1 Put the pineapple, ginger, parsley and vegetables through an electric juicer. Add the aloe vera juice, if using, and stir to combine. Drink immediately or store in the refrigerator up to 1 day. Serve with 1 tablespoon seeds or nuts.

NUTRITIONAL INFORMATION PER SERVING
Protein 8.9g, **Carbohydrates** 33.8g of which sugars 32.8g, **Fat** 8.6g of which saturates 1.2g, **Calories** 250

HEALTH BENEFITS
Aloe vera is a known digestive aid and it is combined here with digestion-supporting gingerroot. Cucumber is hydrating and a source of antioxidants.

Brazil Nut Cream Smoothie

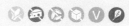

1 Put the nuts in a blender or food processor with
1¾ cups water and process until smooth. Add the
remaining ingredients and process again. Drink
immediately or store in the refrigerator up to 1 day.

SERVES 2, 1 cup each
PREPARATION TIME 5 minutes

scant ½ cup Brazil nuts
1½ cups fresh or frozen strawberries,
    hulled
½ teaspoon vanilla extract
2 teaspoons lecithin granules (optional)

NUTRITIONAL INFORMATION PER SERVING
Protein 5.1g, **Carbohydrates** 6.4g of which sugars 6.4g,
Fat 20.6g of which saturates 5.2g, **Calories** 247

HEALTH BENEFITS
This smoothie contains protein and healthy fats. Brazil nuts are one of the most
concentrated sources of selenium, which is important for protecting cells from damage.

Redbush Apricot Smoothie

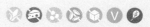

1 Put the tea bag in a measuring jug and pour over 1 cup
boiling water. Leave to soak 10 minutes, then remove
the tea bag and discard. Leave the tea to cool slightly.
2 Put the remaining ingredients into a blender or food
processor and pour the tea over. Process until smooth.
Drink immediately or store in the refrigerator up to
1 day. Serve warm or cold.

SERVES 1, 1 cup
PREPARATION TIME 5 minutes,
    plus 10 minutes soaking

1 redbush (rooibos) tea bag
2 fresh apricots, cut in half and pitted,
    or 4 canned apricot halves, in natural
    juice
heaped ¼ cup cashews
¼ cup ready-to-eat dried apricots

NUTRITIONAL INFORMATION PER SERVING
Protein 9.3g, **Carbohydrates** 22.3g of which sugars 17.7g,
Fat 19.5g of which saturates 3.8g, **Calories** 301

HEALTH BENEFITS
Redbush tea, from the South African rooibos plant, is caffeine-free and low in tannins.
It is also extremely rich in antioxidants, including the flavonoids quercetin and luteolin.

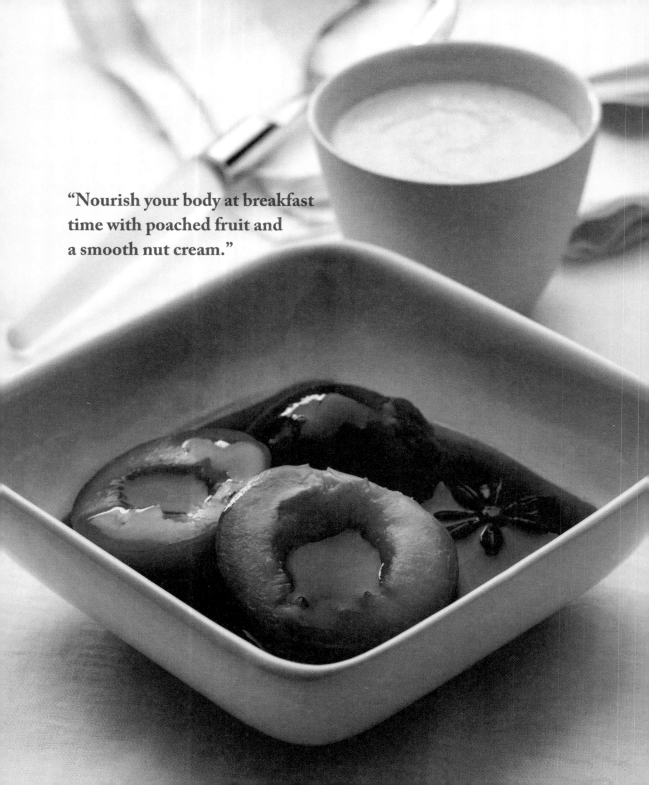

"Nourish your body at breakfast time with poached fruit and a smooth nut cream."

Star Anise-Poached Plums with Ginger-Nut Cream

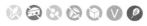

Here, plums are poached in lightly spiced pomegranate juice served with a ginger-nut cream. The plums can be served hot or left to soak in the scented juice and served cold. This is a useful recipe for making in a batch to serve for breakfasts or snacks over two or three days.

1 Put the plums, pomegranate juice, star anise and cinnamon stick in a saucepan. Bring to a boil, then lower the heat and simmer 5 minutes, or until the fruit is just soft. Mix the cornstarch with 1 tablespoon water and add to the pan, stirring until thicker. Leave to cool to develop the flavors.

2 To make the ginger-nut cream, put all the ingredients in a blender or food processor and process until smooth. Add a little water, if necessary.

3 Serve the plums in the syrup either warm or cold with the ginger-nut cream. (Store in the refrigerator up to 3 days.)

SERVES 4
PREPARATION TIME 10 minutes
COOKING TIME 6 minutes, plus
  cooling

6 large or 8 medium red plums, cut in half
  and pitted
1 cup plus 2 tablespoons pure
  pomegranate juice
2 star anise
1 cinnamon stick
2 teaspoons cornstarch or arrowroot

Ginger-nut cream
scant 1 cup cashews
2 tablespoons olive oil or coconut oil
½ cup fresh orange juice
¾-inch piece fresh gingerroot, peeled
  and grated

NUTRITIONAL INFORMATION PER SERVING
Protein 6.3g, **Carbohydrates** 22.6g of which sugars 16.6g, **Fat** 22.7g of which saturates 9.5g, **Calories** 320

HEALTH BENEFITS
Fresh and dried plums (prunes) contain disease-protective phytonutrients, and the high fiber of prunes has a mild laxative effect, aiding bowel function and regularity. Plums are rich in phenols and vitamin C, which can assist with the absorption of iron. Vitamin C is needed in the body to make healthy tissue and support the immune system. The ginger-nut cream provides protein and healthy fats, with the addition of fresh ginger, which helps to support the digestion and ease the symptoms of nausea.

SERVES 8
PREPARATION TIME 10 minutes
COOKING TIME 50 minutes

1½ cups rolled oats

scant ½ cup almonds, chopped

scant ½ cup Brazil nuts, chopped

2 tablespoons chia seeds (optional)

4 tablespoons shelled hempseed

scant ½ cup sunflower seeds

scant ½ cup pumpkin seeds

scant ½ cup sesame seeds

1 tablespoon xylitol or ½ teaspoon stevia
   (optional)

2 tablespoons olive oil or melted coconut
   oil

1 pear, chopped

1 teaspoon cinnamon

½ teaspoon ground ginger

4 tablespoons apple juice

½ cup dried unsweetened berries
   of your choice

⅓ cup goji berries

Mixed Seed Granola

The omega-3 fats in this protein- and nutrient-dense crunchy cereal have been preserved through baking the granola in a low oven. Serve the granola for breakfast with yogurt or milk, or a milk alternative, or use as a snack or topping for fruit dishes.

1 Heat the oven to 315°F and line a cookie sheet with baking parchment. Put the oats, nuts and seeds in a bowl and mix thoroughly. Put the remaining ingredients, except the berries, into a blender or food processor and process until smooth.

2 Pour the wet mixture over the oats, and combine thoroughly with your hands to make sure the oats, nuts and seeds are evenly coated.

3 Spread the mixture onto the prepared cookie sheet. Bake 45 to 50 minutes until golden and crisp. Leave the granola to cool, then stir in the dried berries. Serve. (Store in an airtight container 1 to 2 weeks.)

NUTRITIONAL INFORMATION PER SERVING

Protein 11.3g, **Carbohydrates** 24.4g of which sugars 11g, **Fat** 27.2g of which saturates 5.6g, **Calories** 387

HEALTH BENEFITS

Shelled hempseed are easily digestible and a complete protein source. They also contain high amounts of fatty acids and fiber, trace minerals and vitamin E. The Brazil nuts are selenium rich, and the sunflower and pumpkin seeds are plentiful in omega-6 essential fats.

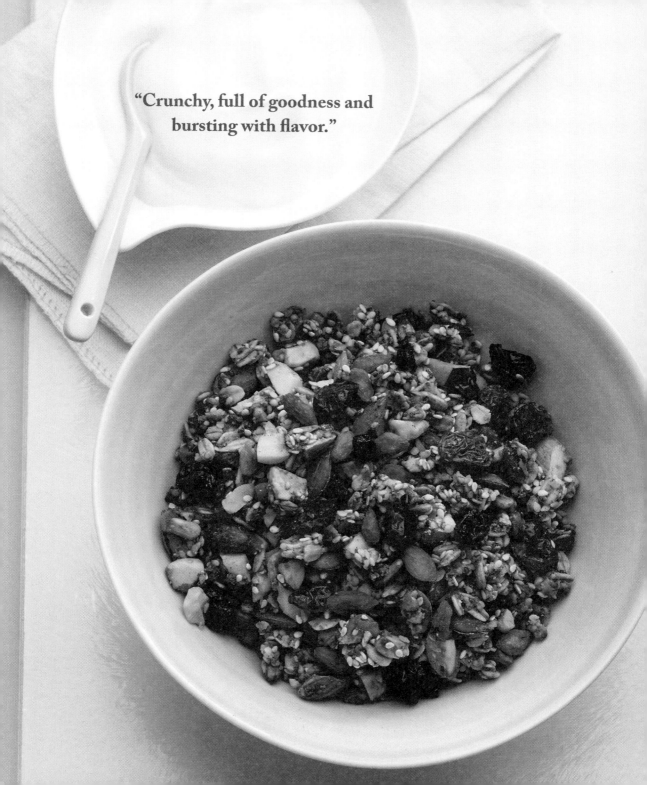

"Crunchy, full of goodness and bursting with flavor."

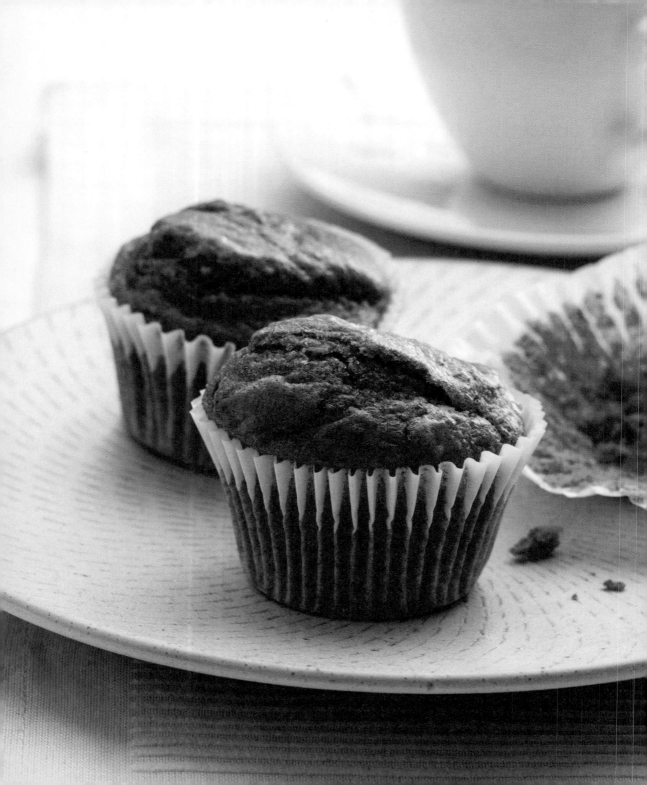

Flaxseed, Apricot & Cinnamon Muffins

These muffins, sweetened with fruit, are rich in soluble fiber thanks to the addition of ground flaxseed. Choose them for a breakfast treat or a healthy snack to keep your energy levels high throughout the day.

MAKES 10
PREPARATION TIME 15 minutes
COOKING TIME 25 minutes, plus cooling

1 Heat the oven to 350°F. Line 10 cups on a muffin pan with paper cases or grease the cups. Into a large bowl, sift together the flour, baking powder, baking soda, salt and cinnamon. Tip in any bran left in the sifter, then stir in the xylitol and flaxseed.

2 Mix together the oil, juice, yogurt and eggs. Add the liquid mixture to the flour mixture and beat with a wooden spoon to make a smooth, thick batter.

3 Stir in the apricots and ginger. Fill each muffin cup about three-quarters full. Bake 20 to 25 minutes until a skewer inserted into the middle of each muffn comes out clean. Leave the muffins to cool for a few minutes before transferring to a wire rack to cool completely before serving. (Store in the refrigerator up to 3 days or freeze up to 1 month.)

4 tablespoons olive oil, plus extra for greasing, if needed
scant 2 cups wholewheat flour or gluten-free flour mix
2 teaspoons baking powder
1 teaspoon baking soda
a pinch sea salt
1½ teaspoons cinnamon
2 tablespoons xylitol
3 tablespoons ground flaxseed
½ cup apple juice
1 cup plain yogurt or soy yogurt
3 eggs
½ cup ready-to-eat dried apricots, chopped
¾-inch piece fresh gingerroot, peeled and grated

NUTRITIONAL INFORMATION PER MUFFIN
Protein 5.7g, **Carbohydrates** 26.8g of which sugars 8.9g, **Fat** 5g of which saturates 1.9g, **Calories** 173

HEALTH BENEFITS
Dried apricots contain soluble fiber to help bowel health. Their high beta-carotene content is converted by the body into vitamin A, which is a powerful antioxidant, quenching free-radical damage to cells and tissues and supporting immune health. Fresh gingerroot is a warming spice frequently used to support digestion and calm the feelings of nausea. Ground cinnamon helps to balance blood sugar levels.

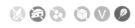

Date & Lucuma Cocoa Bars

MAKES 16

PREPARATION TIME 15 minutes,
plus 10 minutes soaking and at least
1 hour chilling

6 pitted dried dates
heaped 1 cup pecans
1 cup walnut pieces
¼ cup unsweetened cocoa powder
or cacao powder
4 tablespoons shelled hempseed
½ cup lucuma powder
2 tablespoons chia seeds or ground
flaxseed
zest and juice of 1 lemon
4½ tablespoons cashew or almond nut
butter

Lucuma powder is made from a nutrient-dense fruit from Peru, which is traditionally used in ice creams and desserts, and has a maple syrup flavor. Enjoy these healthy raw bars for breakfast or as a snack, straight from the refrigerator, or in a lunch box, although they will be a little softer when eaten at room temperature.

1 Soak the dates in hot water for 10 minutes, then drain and set aside. Line a shallow 8-inch square baking pan with baking parchment. Put the nuts in a blender or food processor and process until very finely ground. Transfer to a bowl and stir in the cocoa powder, hempseed, lucuma powder and chia seeds.

2 Put the dates and lemon zest and juice into the blender or food processor with the nut butter and process until a thick paste forms. Add to the bowl and use your hands to combine all the ingredients into a soft dough.

3 Press the mixture into the prepared pan. Put into the refrigerator and chill 1 to 2 hours until firm, or freeze 1 hour. Cut into bars to serve. (Store, individually wrapped, in the refrigerator up to 1 week or freeze up to 1 month.)

NUTRITIONAL INFORMATION PER BAR
Protein 4.4g, **Carbohydrates** 11.6g of which sugars 6.7g, **Fat** 14.3g of which saturates 1.6g, **Calories** 194

HEALTH BENEFITS
Dates are a great way to add a natural sweetness to dishes, and their soluble fiber slows down the release of sugars in the body to keep you energized for longer. Lucuma is a useful low-glycemic, natural sweetener. It also provides fiber, vitamins and minerals, including beta-carotene, niacin (B3) and iron.

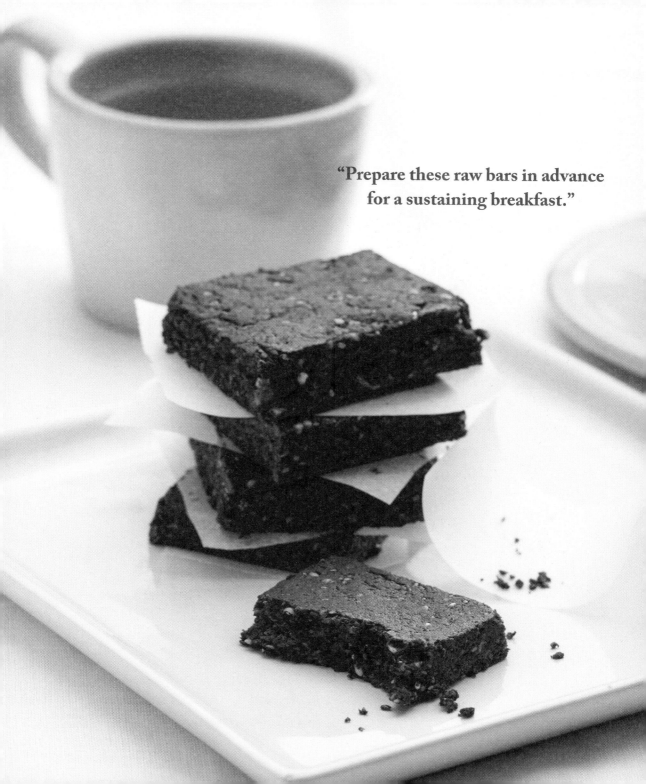

"Prepare these raw bars in advance for a sustaining breakfast."

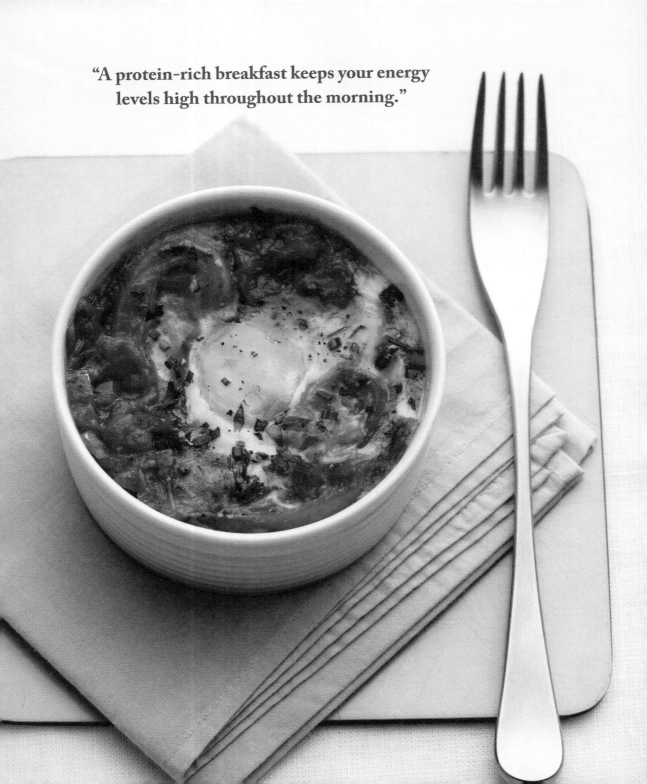

"A protein-rich breakfast keeps your energy levels high throughout the morning."

Spanish Baked Eggs

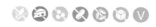

This rustic Spanish-inspired breakfast or brunch-style dish combines antioxidant-rich bell peppers and tomatoes with herbs. It can be mostly prepared in advance—just crack in the eggs when ready to cook. Although the recipe calls for one egg per person, you can add more eggs or a drained and rinsed can of chickpeas to the vegetables.

SERVES 4
PREPARATION TIME 10 minutes
COOKING TIME 20 minutes

2 tablespoons olive oil
1 red onion, finely chopped
1 red bell pepper, seeded and cut
    into strips
1 yellow bell pepper, seeded and cut
    into strips
2 garlic cloves, crushed
½ teaspoon harissa paste, or to taste
½ teaspoon smoked paprika
1 can (15-oz.) crushed tomatoes
2 tablespoons lemon juice
1 tablespoon chopped parsley leaves,
    plus extra to serve
1 tablespoon chopped chives, plus extra
    to serve
4 eggs
freshly ground black pepper

1 Heat the oven to 315°F. Heat the olive oil in a skillet, ideally ovenproof, over low heat and add the onion, peppers, garlic and spices. Cook over low heat 10 minutes, stirring, or until the peppers are soft.

2 Add the tomatoes and simmer 1 to 2 minutes until the sauce is thick. Stir in the lemon juice and scatter the herbs over.

3 If necessary, transfer the vegetables to a shallow baking dish or individual ramekins. Make 4 indents into the mixture, or one for each ramekin, and crack in the eggs. Season with pepper. Bake 6 to 8 minutes until the whites are fully set but the yolks are still a little runny. Serve hot, sprinkled with herbs. (Store in the refrigerator up to 1 day.)

NUTRITIONAL INFORMATION PER SERVING
Protein 8.7g, **Carbohydrates** 9.9g of which sugars 8.9g, **Fat** 10.5g of which saturates 2.3g, **Calories** 169

HEALTH BENEFITS
Garlic contains potent antimicrobial and anticancer phytonutrients. Bell peppers, and particularly the red ones, are among the best sources of vitamin C, which strengthens the immune cells. There is about 250mg vitamin C in a large red bell pepper. The folic acid in the egg yolks is important for the replication of DNA and also protects the DNA during radiotherapy.

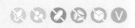

Turkish Breakfast

SERVES 2
PREPARATION TIME 5 minutes
COOKING TIME 15 minutes

3 vine-ripened tomatoes, cut in half
1 zucchini, thickly sliced on the diagonal
2 tablespoons olive oil
1 garlic clove, finely chopped
2 teaspoons chopped oregano
2 eggs
½ cup pitted ripe olives
heaped ⅓ cup crumbled feta cheese
sea salt and freshly ground black pepper

Pitted ripe olives add an accent to this summery, filling dish of Mediterranean roasted tomatoes and zucchini flavored with oregano and garlic. Feta cheese and egg provide protein to accompany the vegetables. It makes an ideal late-morning breakfast. Serve with two eggs per person, if you are avoiding dairy.

1 Heat the oven to 350°F. Put the tomatoes, cut side up, into a baking dish and add the zucchini. Drizzle the oil over and scatter the garlic and oregano over the top. Season with salt and pepper. Roast 15 minutes, or until the vegetables are soft.

2 Meanwhile, pour water into a skillet to a depth of 1 inch. Bring to a boil, then reduce to a simmer. Break the eggs into the water and poach 6 to 8 minutes until the whites are firm but the yolk is a little runny. Toss the olives and cheese into the vegetables, then serve with the poached eggs. (Store in the refrigerator up to 1 day.)

NUTRITIONAL INFORMATION PER SERVING
Protein 13.3g, **Carbohydrates** 4.6g of which sugars 4.5g, **Fat** 19.9g of which saturates 7g, **Calories** 251

HEALTH BENEFITS
Eggs are an economical way to boost your protein intake. One egg contains about 6g complete high-quality protein. Eggs are also a useful source of choline—the key component of many fat-containing structures in cell membranes, making it particularly important for brain function and health.

Sardines with Roasted Tomatoes

Oven-roasting the tomatoes intensifies their sweet flavor, as well as contributing to the nutritional value of this ultrahealthy breakfast choice. Serve with sourdough or rye bread.

1 Heat the oven to 375°F. Stir the garlic into the olive oil.
2 Put the tomatoes on a baking tray and pour the garlic-flavored oil over. Season with salt and pepper. Roast 10 minutes, or until the tomatoes are soft but still holding their shape.
3 Add the spinach leaves and lemon juice and gently stir into the tomatoes, then roast 5 minutes longer. Sprinkle the pine nuts over and serve with the sardines. If you prefer, however, the sardines can be added to the dish with the spinach for the final 5 minutes cooking. (Store in the refrigerator up to 1 day.)

SERVES 4
PREPARATION TIME 5 minutes
COOKING TIME 15 minutes

2 garlic cloves, crushed
2 tablespoons olive oil or melted coconut oil
1½ cups cherry tomatoes
7 ounces baby leaf spinach
1 teaspoon lemon juice
scant ½ cup pine nuts or sunflower seeds
8 ounces canned sardines in water or olive oil, drained
sea salt and freshly ground black pepper

NUTRITIONAL INFORMATION PER SERVING
Protein 20.1g, **Carbohydrates** 2.9g of which sugars 2.8g, **Fat** 22.6g of which saturates 4.7g, **Calories** 295

HEALTH BENEFITS
Serving cooked tomatoes with omega-3-rich oily fish helps to facilitate the absorption of lycopene, an important phytonutrient found in tomatoes, which has been shown to be protective against certain forms of cancer. Vitamin- and mineral-rich spinach is a valuable energizing addition to the dish.

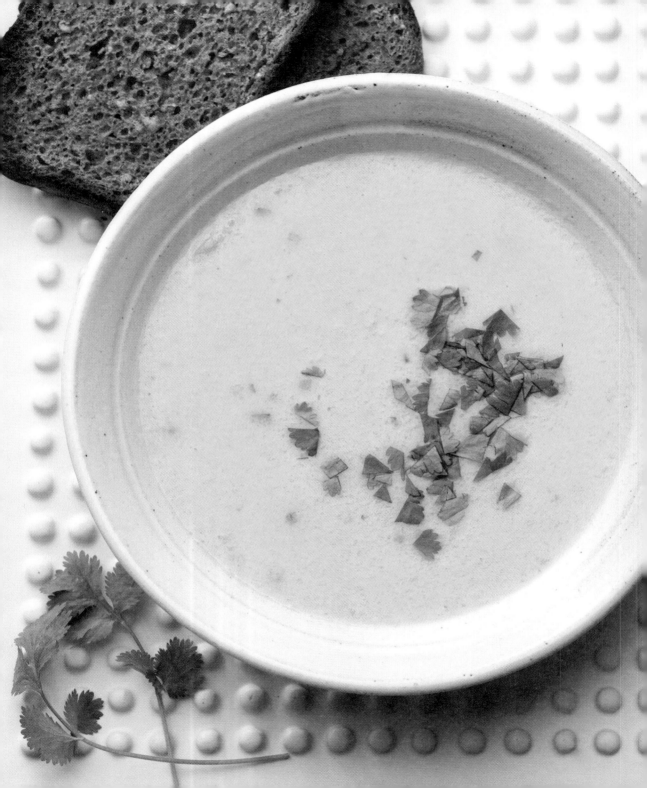

Soups & Light Dishes

When your energy levels and appetite are low, soups and light dishes that are quick and easy to assemble, yet nourishing, are the perfect solution. Simply prepared nutrient-packed broths, or light meat, fish or vegetarian dishes, cram in plenty of foods capable of soothing and healing the body. The recipes in this chapter are a step away from the ordinary, including a sensational dairy-free, creamy Broccoli & Cashew Soup, and a quick-and-easy Sicilian shrimp dish. All the recipes focus on using key ingredients and foods that have been shown to help cancer recovery, promote immune health, reduce inflammation and aid healing, and many can be prepared in advance. If you choose not to eat animal products, several of the recipes can be adapted using vegetable protein.

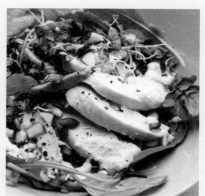

Opposite: Creamy Cauliflower Soup (page 72)
Above: Super-Greens Salad with Chicken (page 77)

SERVES 4

PREPARATION TIME 20 minutes

COOKING TIME 6 minutes

4¼ cups vegetable stock

2 garlic cloves, crushed

½-inch piece fresh gingerroot, peeled
and grated

scant ½ cup cashews

1 teaspoon Thai fish sauce

1 tablespoon apple cider vinegar

1 tablespoon tamari, plus extra
for drizzling

1 pound 2 ounces broccoli, cut into small
pieces

1 tablespoon olive oil or walnut oil

sea salt and freshly ground black pepper

Broccoli & Cashew Soup

This velvety soup can be particularly appealing when your appetite is low or if you're looking for a well-rounded meal in a bowl. It has a hint of Asian flavorings, including the salty, tangy flavor of Thai fish sauce, which complements the flavor of the cashews. Serve this with wholewheat or rye bread.

1 Put the stock, garlic, ginger, cashews, fish sauce, vinegar and tamari into a large saucepan and bring to a boil. Add the broccoli and simmer 2 minutes, or until the broccoli is just tender.

2 Process the soup in a blender or food processor until smooth and thick. Add the oil and process again to combine. Season with salt and pepper. Serve drizzled with a little tamari to taste. (Store in the refrigerator up to 3 days or freeze 1 month.)

NUTRITIONAL INFORMATION PER SERVING

Protein 8.5g, **Carbohydrates** 5.2g of which sugars 2.8g, **Fat** 12.3g of which saturates 2g, **Calories** 167

HEALTH BENEFITS

The combination of broccoli, garlic and gingerroot provides nutrients and phytochemicals that modulate immune function and reduce excess inflammation.

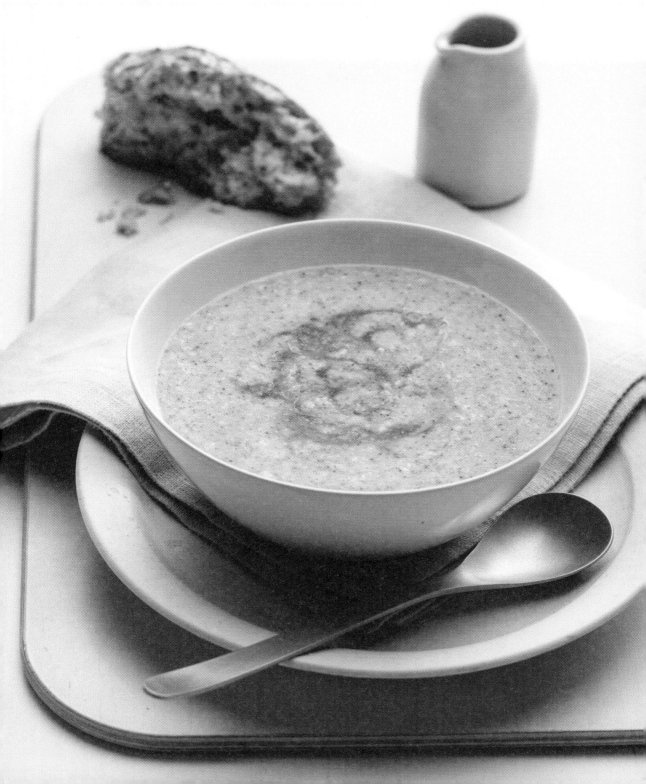

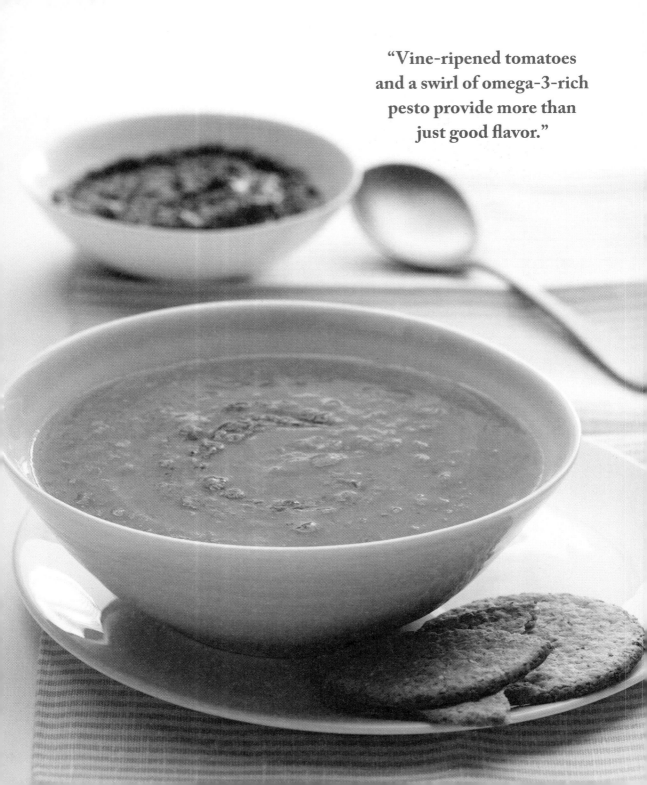

"Vine-ripened tomatoes and a swirl of omega-3-rich pesto provide more than just good flavor."

Garlic & Bean Soup with Pesto

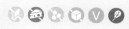

Roasting the garlic and tomatoes creates a naturally sweet and caramelized flavor for this Mediterranean-style soup. The tangy lemon-flavored pesto for the topping can be prepared in advance and refrigerated. You can also thin it down with vegetable stock to make a sauce for drizzling over vegetables and grains. Serve with oat crackers.

1 Heat the oven to 400°F. Put the garlic cloves in a roasting pan, add the olive oil and toss to coat. Roast 15 minutes. Add the tomatoes and roast 10 to 15 minutes longer until the garlic is lightly colored and the tomatoes are soft.
2 Put the garlic, tomatoes, beans and stock into a blender or food processor and process until smooth. Pour into a saucepan and heat gently until warmed through. Add the lemon juice and season with salt and pepper.
3 To make the pumpkin seed pesto, put the nuts and seeds in a food processor and process until finely ground. Add the herbs, garlic, yeast flakes, if using, lemon juice and pinch of salt and process. Drizzle in the oil with the machine running, to create a thick pesto. Serve the soup with a spoonful of pesto. (Store the soup in the refrigerator up to 3 days. Store the pesto in the refrigerator up to 1 week.)

SERVES 4

PREPARATION TIME 10 minutes

COOKING TIME 35 minutes

1 garlic bulb, cloves peeled

2 tablespoons olive oil

1 pound vine-ripened tomatoes, quartered

1 can (15-oz.) borlotti or red kidney beans, drained and rinsed

3 cups vegetable stock

1 tablespoon lemon juice

sea salt and freshly ground black pepper

Pumpkin seed pesto

¼ cup shelled pistachios

scant ¼ cup pumpkin seeds

2 large handfuls basil leaves

1 handful mint leaves

1 garlic clove, crushed

2 tablespoons nutritional yeast flakes (optional)

1 tablespoon lemon juice

2 to 3 tablespoons olive oil or walnut oil

NUTRITIONAL INFORMATION PER SERVING
Protein 5.9g, **Carbohydrates** 13.7g of which sugars 5.5g, **Fat** 3.9g of which saturates 0.5g, **Calories** 116

HEALTH BENEFITS
Tomatoes have a plentiful supply of antioxidants and phytonutrients, which are protective against certain forms of cancer. One, alpha-tomatine, has been linked to prostate cancer prevention, and the carotenoid lycopene might help protect against breast cancer. The pesto is packed with essential omega-3 fats, zinc from the pumpkin seeds and mint to aid digestion.

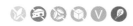

Creamy Cauliflower Soup

SERVES 4
PREPARATION TIME 10 minutes
COOKING TIME 20 minutes

1 tablespoon olive oil or coconut oil
1 onion, finely chopped
3 garlic cloves, roughly chopped
1 red chili, seeded and finely chopped
   (optional)
½ teaspoon turmeric
1 large head cauliflower, cut into florets
1¾ cups canned coconut milk
2½ cups vegetable stock
2 teaspoons tamari
freshly ground black pepper
1 handful cilantro leaves, chopped,
   to serve

A soothing, dairy-free soup with a coconut base and
a little spicy kick from garlic and chili. This soup can
be prepared in advance and reheated. Serve with toasted
wholegrain rye or pumpernickel bread.

1 Heat the oil in a large saucepan over medium heat and fry
   the onion, garlic, chili, if using, and turmeric 5 minutes.
   Add the cauliflower florets and stir to coat in the oil.
2 Pour in the coconut milk, stock and tamari. Bring
   to a boil, then lower the heat and simmer 15 minutes,
   or until the cauliflower is soft. Season to taste with pepper.
3 Process the soup in a blender or food processor until
   smooth. Serve sprinkled with chopped cilantro leaves.
   (Store in the refrigerator up to 3 days or freeze 1 month.)

NUTRITIONAL INFORMATION PER SERVING
Protein 4.7g, **Carbohydrate** 10.7g of which sugars 9.3g, **Fat** 3.8g of which saturates 2.4g, **Calories** 95

HEALTH BENEFITS
The compound curcumin, present in turmeric, has cancer-protective, anti-inflammatory properties, and the chili contains capsaicin,
also known for its anticancer properties. Cauliflower is a cruciferous vegetable that is rich in phytonutrients called glucosinolates, which
can help to activate detoxification enzymes and reduce the toxic burden on the body. It is rich in antioxidants, including vitamin C,
manganese and phytonutrients, as well as vitamin K known for its anti-inflammatory properties.

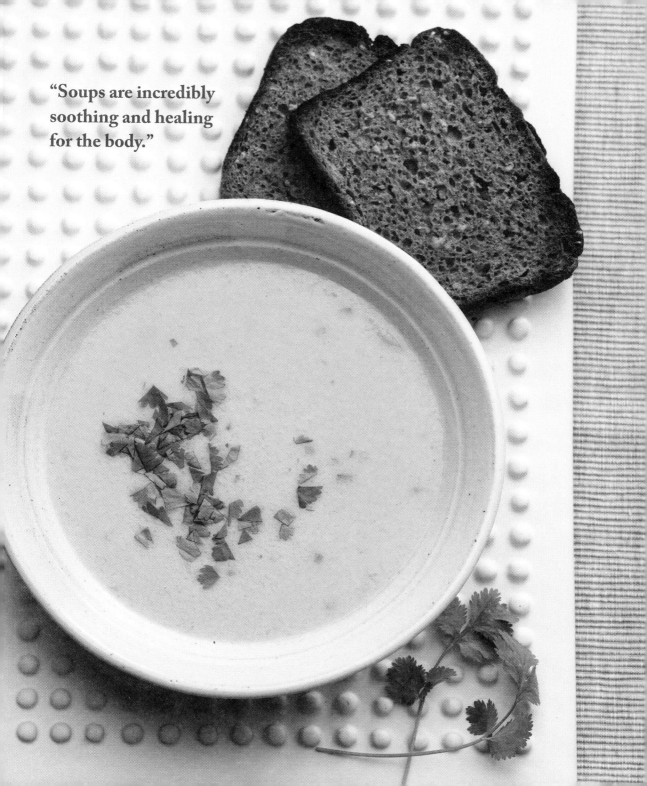

"Soups are incredibly soothing and healing for the body."

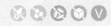

Bell Pepper Bisque with Chili Cream

SERVES 4
PREPARATION TIME 10 minutes
COOKING TIME 25 minutes,
  plus cooling and chilling

3 red bell peppers, halved and seeded
1 tablespoon olive oil or coconut oil
1 red onion, finely chopped
1 garlic clove, crushed
a pinch crushed chilies (optional)
2½ cups vegetable stock
1 can (15-oz.) cannellini beans, drained
  and rinsed

Chili cream
scant ½ cup Greek yogurt
1 red chili, seeded and finely chopped
2 tablespoons roughly chopped basil
  leaves

Cannellini beans add protein to this chilled summer soup topped with a little chili-infused yogurt, although the chili can be omitted if you prefer. The soup is also excellent served hot. Serve with sourdough bread or oat crackers.

1 Heat the broiler. Put the peppers cut side down on a cookie sheet and broil until the skin is charred all over. Transfer to a bowl, cover with plastic wrap and leave to cool 10 minutes. Peel off the skins and chop the flesh.
2 Heat the olive oil in a large saucepan over low heat and fry the onion and garlic 3 to 4 minutes until soft. Add the peppers and chilies, if using, and stir to combine.
3 Pour in the stock and beans and bring to a boil. Simmer, covered, 10 minutes. Process the soup in a blender or food processor, then pass it through a strainer. Cover and chill until required (or keep warm if serving hot).
4 To make the chili cream, put the yogurt, chili and basil into a food processor and pulse briefly to combine—leave some visible flakes of chili and basil. Serve the soup topped with a spoonful of the chili cream. (Store in the refrigerator up to 3 days or freeze 1 month.)

NUTRITIONAL INFORMATION PER SERVING
Protein 4.8g, **Carbohydrates** 13.6g of which sugars 6.5g, **Fat** 3.5g of which saturates 2.4g, **Calories** 104

HEALTH BENEFITS
Cannellini beans provide protein, as well as soluble fiber to support digestive health. Bell peppers are an excellent source of vitamin C and they also provide cancer-protective phytochemicals, such as lycopene and beta-carotene (the precursor for vitamin A).

Asian Turkey Patties with Dipping Sauce

The Asian flavors in these little patties make them especially tempting if your appetite is flat. The patties are rich in protein and B vitamins to perk up flagging energy levels, and the dipping sauce, made with yogurt, ginger and mint, can be helpful for settling digestive upsets. Serve with a mixed salad or steamed greens.

1 To make the sauce, put all the ingredients into a blender or food processor and blend briefly to combine. Chill until required.

2 Put the turkey into the blender or food processor with the fish sauce, tamari, ginger, onion and garlic. Blend to form a coarse puree. Transfer to a bowl, then cover and chill 20 minutes.

3 With damp hands, shape the mixture into 8 patties. Heat the olive oil in a skillet over medium heat and brown the patties in batches 3 to 4 minutes on each side until cooked through. Serve the patties with the dipping sauce. (Store in the refrigerator up to 3 days or freeze, uncooked, 1 month.)

SERVES 2
PREPARATION TIME 15 minutes, plus chilling
COOKING TIME 16 minutes

9 ounces boneless, skinless turkey breast, chopped
2 tablespoons Thai fish sauce
1 tablespoon tamari
½-inch piece fresh gingerroot, peeled and grated
½ red onion, finely chopped
1 garlic clove, crushed
1 tablespoon olive oil or coconut oil

Dipping sauce
¾ cup plus 2 tablespoons Greek yogurt or soy yogurt
2 green chilies, seeded and chopped (optional)
1 large handful mint leaves, chopped
1½-inch piece fresh gingerroot, peeled and grated
sea salt and freshly ground black pepper

NUTRITIONAL INFORMATION PER SERVING
Protein 36.6g, **Carbohydrates** 16.6g of which sugars 14.9g, **Fat** 2.2g of which saturates 1g, **Calories** 225

HEALTH BENEFITS
Lean turkey meat is high in protein and is served here with ginger to aid digestion. The capsaicin in chilies gives them their characteristic pungency and it is a potent inhibitor of substance P, a neuropeptide associated with inflammatory processes. Studies also suggest it might stop the spread of prostate cancer cells and lessen the expression of prostate-specific antigen (PSA).

"A blend of natural flavors
invigorates and nourishes your whole body."

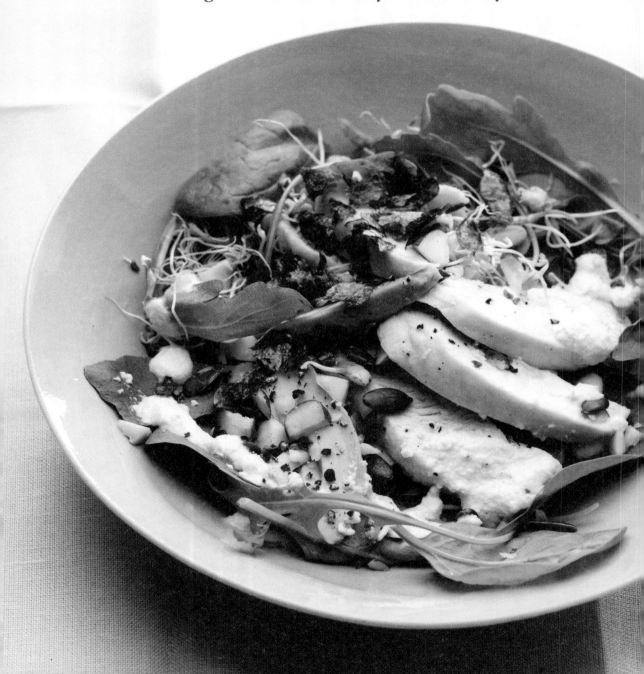

Super-Greens Salad with Chicken

Try this tangy, peppery and nutrient-dense green salad that is packed with vitamins, minerals, protein and healthy fats. The inclusion of nuts and seeds adds crunch and provides the essential minerals magnesium, manganese, iron, zinc and selenium. The roasted chicken, for additional protein, can be omitted or replaced with canned beans or chickpeas, drained and rinsed.

1 To make the dressing, soak the cashews in water 20 minutes, then drain. Put them into a blender or food processor with all the other dressing ingredients. Add ½ cup water, season lightly with pepper and process until a light pouring consistency forms. Add a little more water, if necessary.

2 In a large bowl, toss together the arugula, spinach, watercress, alfalfa and bean sprouts. Toss in a little of the dressing to just coat the leaves, if you like.

3 Slice the chicken. Serve the salad with the avocado slices, nuts, seeds and the chicken slices, and the nori sheet crumbled over the top. Drizzle a little extra dressing over. (Store, without dressing, in the refrigerator up to 2 days.)

SERVES 4

PREPARATION TIME 10 minutes, plus 20 minutes soaking

4 ounces each arugula leaves, baby spinach leaves and watercress leaves
2 cups alfalfa sprouts
heaped ½ cup mung bean sprouts
2 boneless, skinless roasted chicken breast halves
1 ripe avocado, sliced
scant ½ cup Brazil nuts, roughly chopped
scant ¼ cup pumpkin seeds
1 nori sheet

Nut dressing
scant 1 cup cashews
1 garlic clove
zest and juice of 1 lime
2 teaspoons spirulina or chlorella powder (optional)
2 teaspoons nutritional yeast flakes (optional)
freshly ground black pepper

NUTRITIONAL INFORMATION PER SERVING (WITH 1 TABLESPOON DRESSING)
Protein 25.1g, **Carbohydrates** 4.2g of which sugars 1.5g, **Fat** 24.2g of which saturates 5.4g, **Calories** 335

HEALTH BENEFITS
Bitter leafy greens, such as arugula and watercress, are useful for stimulating digestive secretions and are packed with protective antioxidants. The use of the optional green superfood powders—spirulina and chlorella—in the dressing is an excellent way to add more amino acids (protein building blocks), vitamins and minerals to your diet.

SERVES 4
PREPARATION TIME 15 minutes
COOKING TIME 15 minutes

14 ounces lean ground lamb
1 garlic clove, crushed
1 red onion, grated
1 tablespoon olive oil or coconut oil
   (optional)
sea salt and freshly ground black pepper

Wasabi mayonnaise
5 ounces silken tofu, cubed
3 tablespoons olive oil or flaxseed oil
1 tablespoon lemon juice
1 teaspoon xylitol or ½ teaspoon stevia
a pinch matcha green tea powder
   (optional)
1 teaspoon wasabi powder

Japanese Lamb Burgers with Wasabi Mayo

A tangy wasabi mayonnaise accompanies these quick-and-easy burgers. The burgers can be frozen uncooked, making them ideal for cooking when you don't feel like preparing food. Either fry or broil them and serve them with a green salad or steamed vegetables.

1 Put the lamb into a large bowl and add the garlic and onion. Season. Using your hands, mix well, then shape the mixture into 8 balls and press into burger shapes.

2 If frying the burgers, heat the oil in a skillet over medium heat, then fry the burgers 5 minutes on each side, or until cooked through. Alternatively, heat the broiler. Put the burgers on a foil-lined baking tray and broil 6 to 7 minutes on each side until cooked through, but not overbrown.

3 To make the mayonnaise, put all the ingredients into a blender or food processor and process until smooth. Add a little water, if it seems too thick. Season the burgers lightly with pepper and serve with the mayonnaise. (The uncooked burgers can be frozen up to 1 month.)

NUTRITIONAL INFORMATION PER SERVING
Protein 22.4g, **Carbohydrates** 2.7g of which sugars 2.2g, **Fat** 23.9g of which saturates 9.3g, **Calories** 314

HEALTH BENEFITS
Grass-fed lamb is a good source of omega-3 fats. It is also rich in protein, antioxidants, selenium and zinc for immune support, and B vitamins, which are important for energy. Distinctively flavored Japanese wasabi is traditionally used for its flavor and included here for its antimicrobial, anticancer and anti-inflammatory benefits.

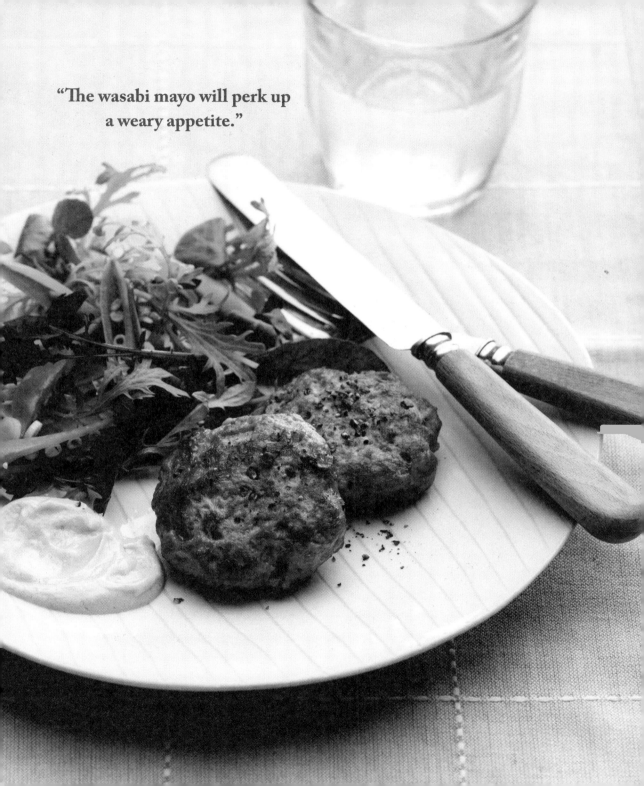

"The wasabi mayo will perk up a weary appetite."

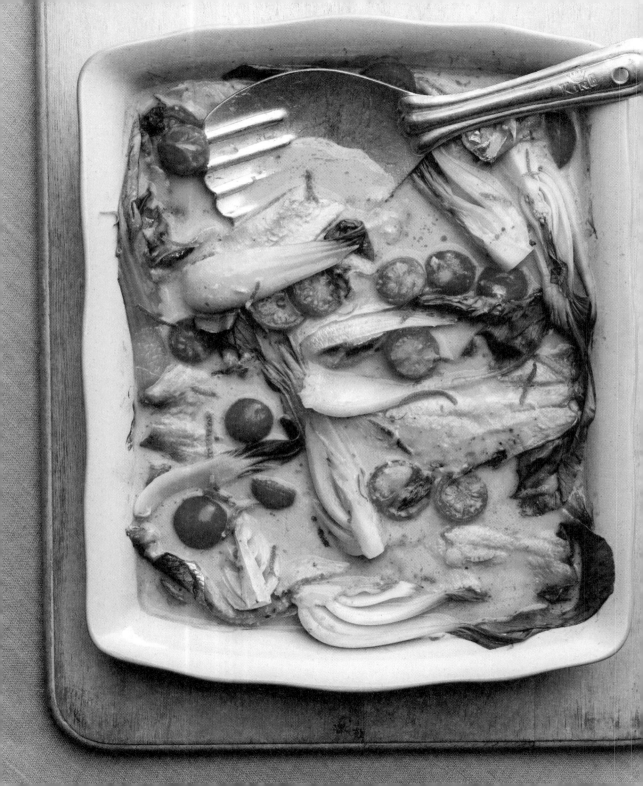

Coconut- & Lime- Baked Sardines

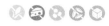

When you feel low in energy this dish will appeal, because it requires minimal preparation and is full of flavor. Sardines are inexpensive and full of nutrients, and adding greens to the mix makes this a convenient one-pot meal that scores on all the healthy points. You can also make this with mackerel fillets.

SERVES 4
PREPARATION TIME 10 minutes
COOKING TIME 25 minutes

1¾ cups canned coconut milk
1 tablespoon cornstarch
2 teaspoons Thai red curry paste
zest and juice of 1 lime
1 teaspoon turmeric
6 tablespoons vegetable stock or water
8 sardines or 4 small mackerel, dressed
  and filleted
2 bok choy, cut into quarters
12 cherry tomatoes, cut in half
sea salt and freshly ground black pepper

1 Heat the oven to 350°F. Mix a little of the coconut milk with the cornstarch to make a smooth paste. In a saucepan, mix together the remaining coconut milk with the cornstarch paste, curry paste, lime zest and juice, turmeric and stock and warm slowly, stirring continuously. Continue to stir until the mixture is thick. Season with salt and pepper.

2 Put the sardines, skin side down, into a large, shallow baking dish and add the bok choy. Pour the coconut sauce over and scatter the tomatoes between the sardines. Bake 20 minutes, or until the sardines are cooked through. Serve. (This is best eaten fresh but can be stored in the refrigerator up to 1 day.)

NUTRITIONAL INFORMATION PER SERVING
Protein 43.5g, **Carbohydrates** 15.1g of which sugars 8.4g, **Fat** 20.2g of which saturates 5.7g, **Calories** 413

HEALTH BENEFITS
Sardines are an abundant source of anti-inflammatory omega-3 fats, plus protein, to help maintain muscle mass and facilitate healing, as well as containing vitamin D, calcium and selenium.

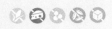

Sicilian Shrimp

SERVES 4
PREPARATION TIME 15 minutes,
    plus 1 hour or overnight marinating
COOKING TIME 3 minutes

24 raw jumbo shrimp, shelled
1 teaspoon olive oil or coconut oil

Fresh herb dressing
2 tablespoons capers, rinsed
1 canned anchovy fillet
2 garlic cloves
a pinch crushed chilies (optional)
1 handful each cilantro leaves, mint leaves
    and parsley leaves
3 tablespoons balsamic vinegar
6 tablespoons olive oil
sea salt and freshly ground black pepper

Roasted bell pepper salad
3 roasted red bell peppers from a jar,
    drained and sliced into strips
1 red onion, finely chopped
2 tablespoons capers, rinsed
8 pitted ripe olives, cut in half

Succulent jumbo shrimp are marinated in a fresh herb dressing and served with a simple roasted bell pepper salad in this quick-to-prepare meal that's rich in protein. Marinating the shrimp in the dressing heightens their flavor. The salad and dressing can also be eaten without the shrimp for a light and healthy meal or snack.

1 To make the dressing, put all the ingredients into a mini food processor and pulse to combine to a coarse texture.
2 Put the shrimp into a shallow dish and pour over half the dressing. Cover and leave to marinate in the refrigerator at least 1 to 2 hours, or overnight.
3 Heat the olive oil in a skillet over medium heat. Add the shrimp with their dressing and stir 2 to 3 minutes until cooked though and pink.
4 Mix all the salad ingredients together in a bowl. Serve the salad topped with the shrimp and with the remaining dressing drizzled over. (Store, without dressing, in the refrigerator up to 2 days.)

NUTRITIONAL INFORMATION PER SERVING
Protein 12.8g, **Carbohydrates** 5.4g of which sugars 4.9g, **Fat** 25.6g of which saturates 4.3g, **Calories** 306

HEALTH BENEFITS
Shrimp are a good source of omega-3 fats, selenium and B vitamins. Docosahexaenoic acid (DHA), an omega-3 fatty acid found in shrimp and cold-water fish, has been shown to reduce the size of tumors and enhance the positive effects of certain chemotherapy drugs while limiting their side effects.

Pan-Fried Squid, Red Cabbage & Walnuts

Serve this warm, crunchy salad as an alternative for coleslaw. Red cabbage is a nutrient-rich cruciferous vegetable and, combined with apple, nuts and cherries, makes a colorful and healthy dish. The salad is also nourishing served without the squid.

1 Lightly toast the walnuts in a dry skillet over medium heat 1 minute, stirring, then chop them roughly. Set aside. Slit the squid tubes down one side, then open them out and score the inside lightly in a crisscross pattern. Cut into bite-size pieces. Season lightly with salt and pepper.

2 Heat the olive oil in a skillet over medium heat. Add the squid tubes and tentacles and stir-fry 1 to 2 minutes until just cooked. Remove with a slotted spoon and set aside. Add the cabbage, garlic, ginger and chili, if using, and stir-fry 3 minutes to soften the cabbage slightly.

3 Stir in the apples, vinegar, tamari and lime juice and stir 3 to 4 minutes longer until the cabbage is soft but still crunchy. Stir in the squid to warm through. Toss in the herbs and transfer to a bowl. Sprinkle the walnuts and cherries over and season with salt and pepper. Serve.

SERVES 4
PREPARATION TIME 10 minutes
COOKING TIME 10 minutes

½ cup walnut pieces
9 ounces dressed squid, with tentacles reserved
2 tablespoons olive oil or coconut oil
1 small red cabbage, shredded
2 garlic cloves, crushed
½-inch piece fresh gingerroot, peeled and grated
½ red chili, seeded and finely diced (optional)
2 eating apples, grated
3 tablespoons apple cider vinegar
2 tablespoons tamari
1 tablespoon fresh lime juice
2 tablespoons chopped mint leaves
2 tablespoons chopped cilantro leaves
scant ½ cup dried unsweetened cherries
sea salt and freshly ground black pepper

NUTRITIONAL INFORMATION PER SERVING
Protein 13.9g, **Carbohydrates** 22.9g of which sugars 21.6g, **Fat** 16.3g of which saturates 5.3g, **Calories** 291

HEALTH BENEFITS
Seafood, such as squid, provides additional protein, plus the minerals copper, selenium, phosphorus and magnesium. Selenium is particularly important for reducing inflammation. Copper is required by the body for the formation of red blood cells, which help maintain energy levels.

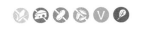

Hoisin Tempeh Skewers

SERVES 4
PREPARATION TIME 5 minutes,
    plus at least 1 hour marinating
COOKING TIME 10 minutes

14 ounces tempeh
3 tablespoons hoisin sauce
2 tablespoons tamari
¾-inch piece fresh gingerroot, peeled
    and grated
1 red chili, seeded and chopped (optional)
1 garlic clove, crushed
3 tablespoons mirin or 1 tablespoon rice
    wine
2 tablespoons vegetable stock or water

Pickled cucumber salad
½ cucumber
1 small red chili, seeded and thinly sliced
    into ribbons (optional)
juice of ½ lime
2 tablespoons rice wine vinegar
2 tablespoons tamari
1 tablespoon toasted nori flakes
2 tablespoons finely chopped cilantro,
    to serve

Nutty-tasting tempeh is a highly nutritious fermented
food made from soybeans. It is rich in protein and fiber,
and makes a sustaining and energizing light dish that
is also suitable for snacking on. It is served here with
a pickled cucumber salad.

1 Pat the tempeh dry and cut it into ¾-inch cubes. Mix
   together the hoisin sauce, tamari, ginger, chili, if using,
   garlic, mirin and stock. Put the tempeh into a shallow dish
   and pour the marinade over. Leave to marinate at least
   1 hour, or overnight.
2 To make the salad, cut the cucumber into long ribbons
   using a vegetable peeler. Put them into a bowl with the
   chili, if using. Mix together the remaining ingredients and
   pour over the cucumber. Leave to marinate 30 minutes.
   Meanwhile, soak 8 wooden skewers in water.
3 Heat the broiler to high. Line a baking tray with baking
   parchment. Thread 4 pieces of tempeh onto each skewer
   and put onto the tray. Broil 8 to 10 minutes until golden,
   turning occasionally and brushing with marinade. Sprinkle
   the cilantro over the salad and serve with the tempeh.
   (Store in the refrigerator up to 2 days.)

NUTRITIONAL INFORMATION PER SERVING
Protein 21.7g, **Carbohydrates** 12.5g of which sugars 2.1g, **Fat** 6.9g of which saturates 0g, **Calories** 210

HEALTH BENEFITS
Tempeh is rich in fiber, antioxidants and naturally occurring isoflavones, including genistein, which has been linked to a lower incidence
of certain cancers, such as prostate. Genistein has been shown to induce the chemicals that block cell cycling, thus preventing the
proliferation of cancerous cells in the prostate.

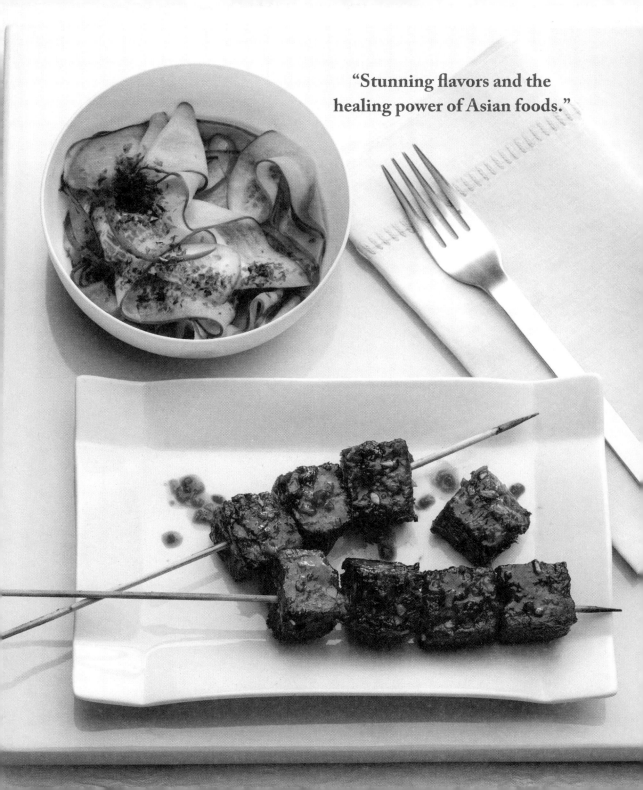

"Stunning flavors and the healing power of Asian foods."

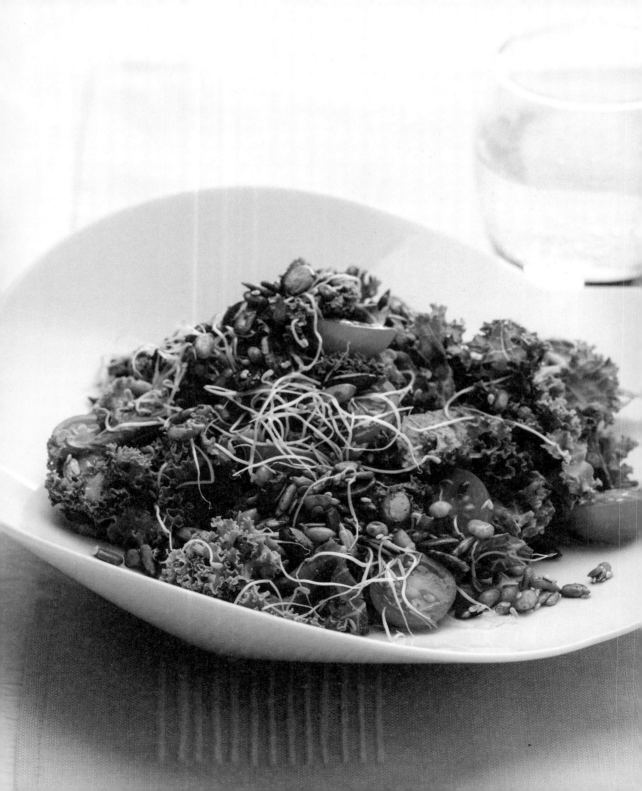

Wilted Kale Salad with Toasted Seeds

This simple, cleansing salad is quick to prepare and ideal for a very light lunch to accompany hard-boiled eggs or feta cheese. The toasted seeds and nuts can also be eaten as a tasty and wholesome snack, so it's worth making up a batch and keeping it in an airtight container ready to eat with a drink of fruit juice or a smoothie.

1 To make the toasted seeds and nuts, put them in a dry skillet over medium heat and lightly toast, stirring, 1 minute. As they begin to color, pour the tamari over and stir to combine. Stir 1 to 2 minutes until crisp. Leave to cool.

2 Put the kale into a large bowl and sprinkle the garlic salt and yeast flakes, if using, over. Massage with your hands to let the kale soften. Put the avocado, lemon juice, cumin, oil and tamari into a blender or food processor and process until smooth. Mix these ingredients into the kale until it is thoroughly coated. Stir in the tomatoes and sprinkle the alfalfa sprouts and toasted seeds and nuts over, then serve. (Store in the refrigerator up to 2 days.)

SERVES 4
PREPARATION TIME 10 minutes
COOKING TIME 3 minutes

3¾ cups roughly chopped kale leaves
1 teaspoon garlic salt
1 tablespoon nutritional yeast flakes (optional)
1 ripe avocado, seeded and peeled
3 tablespoons lemon juice
½ teaspoon ground cumin
1 tablespoon olive oil or flaxseed oil
2 teaspoons tamari
1¼ cups cherry tomatoes, cut in half
1 handful alfalfa sprouts

Toasted seeds and nuts

2 tablespoons pine nuts
6 tablespoons mixed seeds, such as sunflower seeds, pumpkin seeds and hempseed
2 tablespoons tamari

NUTRITIONAL INFORMATION PER SERVING
Protein 9.8g, **Carbohydrates** 7.8g of which sugars 4.8g, **Fat** 24.3g of which saturates 3.1g, **Calories** 289

HEALTH BENEFITS
Kale is a cruciferous super-food rich in glucosinolates, which can play a primary role in protection against many forms of cancer. It is also packed with flavonoids: antioxidants that help lower inflammation and protect against cell damage. (People with thyroid problems should limit their intake of raw cruciferous vegetables, because they can lower the function of the thyroid and reduce metabolism.)

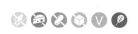

SERVES 4
PREPARATION TIME 15 minutes

½ celery root
2 apples, cored and cut into thin slices
2 fennel bulbs, cut into thin slices
2 tablespoons capers, rinsed and
    finely chopped
8 small gherkins, finely chopped
3 tablespoons chopped parsley leaves,
    plus extra to serve
2 tablespoons chopped mint leaves
sea salt and freshly ground black pepper

Tofu mayonnaise
5 ounces silken tofu
1 tablespoon Dijon mustard
zest and juice of 1 lemon
⅔ cup olive oil or omega-blended oil
    (a combination of flaxseed oil, olive oil,
    hempseed oil)
a little vegetable stock or water, if needed

Celery Root, Apple & Fennel Rémoulade

This dish is dairy-free, and the tofu mayonnaise provides protein, calcium, magnesium and phytoestrogens. To add a little color and additional liver support, include grated raw beets. For extra protein, add a few walnuts or pecans, or serve the salad with meat or fish. Silken tofu, used for the dressing, is a soft tofu suitable for making into sauces and desserts.

1 To make the mayonnaise, put the tofu, mustard and lemon juice into a blender or food processor and switch on. Add the oil in a steady stream to form a thick, creamy sauce. You might need to add a little water or stock to thin it slightly. Stir in the lemon zest and set aside.

2 Cut the celery root into matchstick strips and put into a large bowl with the apples and fennel. Add the capers, gherkins, parsley and mint. Pour the tofu mayonnaise over and mix to combine. Season with salt and pepper and sprinkle with parsley, then serve. (Store in the refrigerator up to 3 days.)

NUTRITIONAL INFORMATION PER SERVING
Protein 4.9g, **Carbohydrates** 6.9g of which sugars 6.5g, **Fat** 37.1g of which saturates 3.5g, **Calories** 407

HEALTH BENEFITS
Fennel is well known for its digestive properties and aids fat digestion by stimulating the gallbladder and increasing the flow of bile. Apples are a good source of pectin, a soluble fiber that assists digestion.

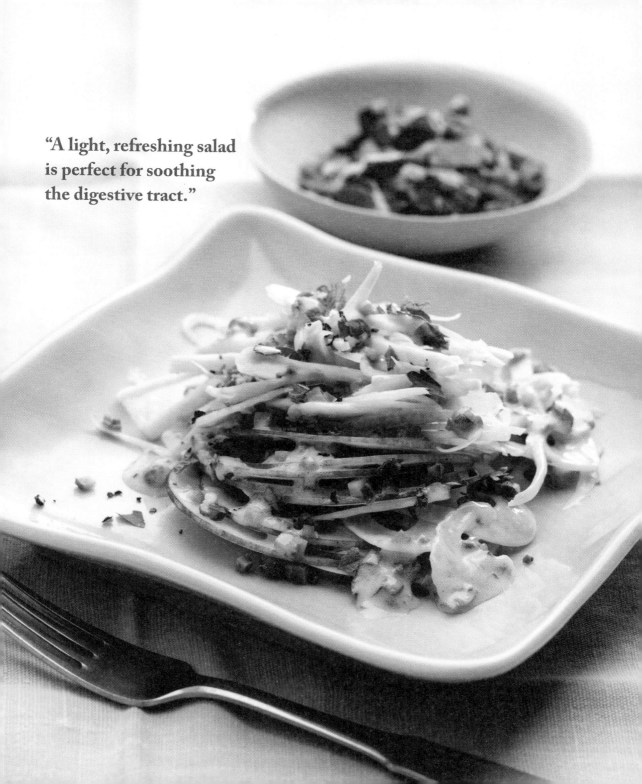

"A light, refreshing salad is perfect for soothing the digestive tract."

Mixed Sea Vegetable & Cucumber Salad

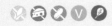

SERVES 4
PREPARATION TIME 10 minutes,
   plus 15 minutes soaking
COOKING TIME 5 minutes

2 ounces mixed dried seaweed
2 cups frozen edamame
   (soybeans)
1 cucumber
7 ounces arugula leaves or a mixture
   of leafy greens
3 scallions, thinly sliced

Lime soy dressing
2 tablespoons olive oil or flaxseed oil
½-inch piece fresh gingerroot, peeled
   and grated
zest and juice of 1 lime
1 tablespoon tamari

Adding sea vegetables to salad is an easy way to increase your intake of iodine, which is typically low in many people's diets and a deficiency has been linked to the development of breast cancer. This Japanese-inspired dish is light and refreshing and can be served with steamed fish or shrimp.

1 Soak the seaweed in water 15 minutes, or according to the package directions, then drain thoroughly. Put the edamame in a steamer and steam over high heat 5 minutes, or until just tender, then drain and refresh under cold water.

2 Cut the cucumber into long strips using a vegetable peeler. Put all the dressing ingredients into a small bowl and whisk well.

3 Toss the arugula, sea vegetables, scallions, cucumber and edamame together in a large bowl, then drizzle the dressing over and toss to coat before serving. (Store, without dressing, in the refrigerator up to 2 days.)

NUTRITIONAL INFORMATION PER SERVING
Protein 11.9g, **Carbohydrates** 4.3g of which sugars 3.2g, **Fat** 10.5g of which saturates 1.2g, **Calories** 163

HEALTH BENEFITS
Sea vegetables, such as dulse, kelp, nori and arame, are rich in trace minerals and sulfur, which might play a role in lowering the risk of estrogen-related cancers, including breast cancer.

Warm Lentil & Bean Salad

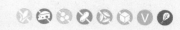

Cannellini beans are creamy in texture and contrast beautifully with the crunchy celery and Puy lentils, and the sweet flavor of roasted tomatoes. You can use canned Puy lentils, if you prefer, for this sustaining salad.

SERVES 4

PREPARATION TIME 10 minutes

COOKING TIME 20 minutes

3 tablespoons olive oil

3 garlic cloves, crushed

1½ cups cherry tomatoes, cut in half

1 cup Puy lentils, rinsed

1 red onion, finely chopped

1 celery stick, finely chopped

1 can (15-oz.) cannellini beans, drained and rinsed

2 tablespoons balsamic vinegar

2 tablespoons finely chopped mint leaves

2 tablespoons finely chopped parsley leaves

sea salt and freshly ground black pepper

1 Heat the oven to 400°F. Mix together 2 tablespoons of the olive oil and all the garlic. Put the cherry tomatoes in a baking dish and drizzle the garlic-flavored oil over. Roast 10 minutes, or until just soft.

2 Meanwhile, put the lentils in a saucepan and add enough water to cover them. Bring to a boil, then simmer 10 to 12 minutes until just cooked. Drain and rinse.

3 Heat the remaining olive oil in a skillet over medium heat and gently fry the onion and celery 2 to 3 minutes until soft. Add the lentils, beans and balsamic vinegar and cook 1 to 2 minutes longer to heat through. Toss in the tomatoes and herbs, and season with salt and pepper. Serve. (Store in the refrigerator up to 3 days.)

NUTRITIONAL INFORMATION PER SERVING

Protein 16.6g, **Carbohydrates** 34.3g of which sugars 5.1g, **Fat** 8.3g of which saturates 2.8g, **Calories** 281

HEALTH BENEFITS

Roasting the tomatoes optimizes the availability of lycopene: a potent antioxidant for helping with cancer recovery. Beans and lentils are a good source of protein, soluble fiber and phytoestrogens, and the garlic has anti-inflammatory properties.

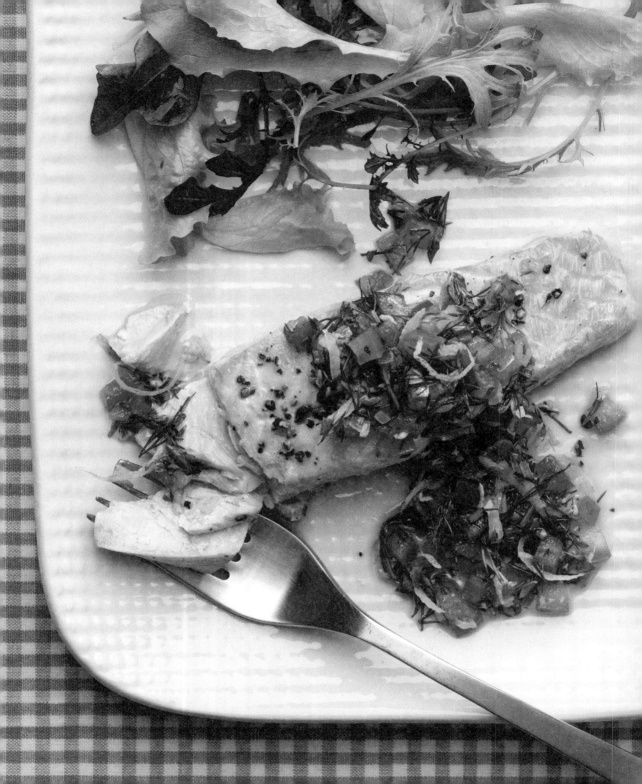

Main Meals

During cancer treatment and recovery there might be times when you crave warming comfort foods that are rich in flavor and also full of nourishing ingredients. In this chapter we have created a selection of appealing, easy-to-assemble main meals to satisfy your appetite while also optimizing nutrition. We focus on using key ingredients to help protect and heal the body, while making sure each meal is tempting in flavor and appearance.

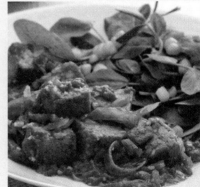

There are new slants on favorites, such as our Mixed Seafood Pie and Turkey & Pistachio Korma, plus more classic Balsamic-Braised Duck, and the more exotic combinations of Chicken and Cashew Stir-Fry and our Tamarind-Spiced Mackerel. Many of the dishes are suitable for preparing in advance or freezing.

Opposite: Salmon with Sauce Vierge (page 104)
Above: Roasted Tempeh with Pipérade Sauce (page 110)

Chicken & Cashew Stir-Fry

SERVES 4
PREPARATION TIME 10 minutes
COOKING TIME 10 minutes

scant ½ cup cashews

1 egg

1 tablespoon cornstarch

1 pound boneless, skinless chicken breast
    halves, sliced

1 tablespoon olive oil or coconut oil

4 scallions, sliced

3 ounces snow peas, trimmed

1 bok choy, leaves separated

1 yellow bell pepper, seeded and sliced
    into strips

1 red bell pepper, seeded and sliced
    into strips

⅔ cup sliced shiitake mushrooms

4 tablespoons chicken stock

juice of 1 lime

2 to 3 tablespoons tamari

2 tablespoons cilantro leaves, chopped

sea salt and freshly ground black pepper

For this super-quick dish, strips of chicken flavored with cilantro and lime are tossed with a colorful medley of vegetables and toasted nuts. Choose organic chicken if possible to reduce your exposure to added hormones and antibiotics. Serve with buckwheat or wholewheat noodles.

1 Lightly toast the nuts in a dry skillet over medium heat 1 minute, stirring, then set aside. Put the egg into a large bowl, add the cornstarch and a pinch of salt and whisk to combine. Add the chicken and coat with the egg mixture.

2 Heat a skillet or wok with the olive oil over medium heat. Stir-fry the chicken 4 to 5 minutes until lightly colored, then remove with a slotted spoon.

3 Add the scallions and stir-fry a few seconds. Add the snow peas, bok choy and peppers and stir-fry 1 minute longer, or until just soft. Add the chicken, mushrooms, stock, lime juice and tamari to taste. Simmer 1 minute longer, or until the mushrooms are soft. Stir in the nuts and cilantro, then season with salt and pepper. Serve. (Store in the refrigerator up to 3 days.)

NUTRITIONAL INFORMATION PER SERVING
Protein 34.9g, **Carbohydrates** 17g of which sugars 8.2g, **Fat** 12.9g of which saturates 4.2g, **Calories** 323

HEALTH BENEFITS
Chicken is an energizing food, rich in B vitamins and protein and low in saturated fats. It is an excellent source of the cancer-protective B vitamin, niacin, which helps protect components of DNA.

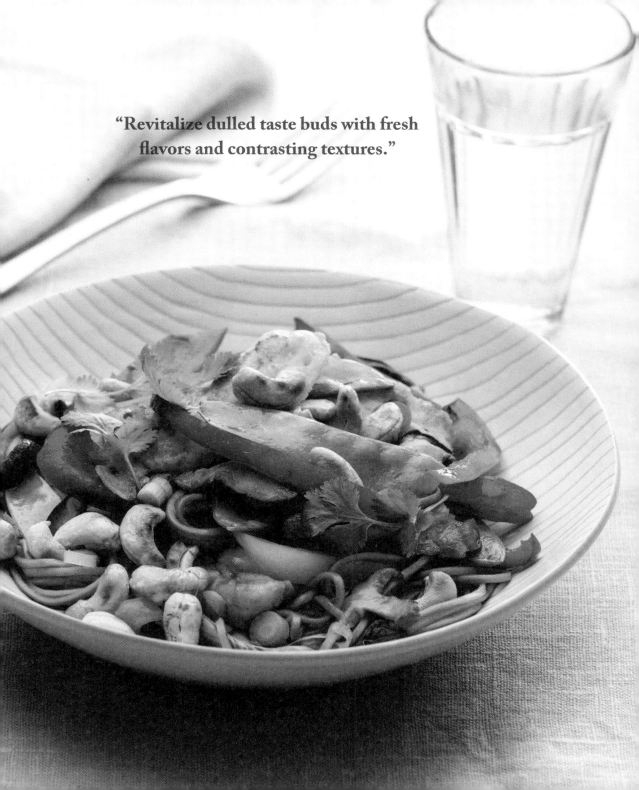

"Revitalize dulled taste buds with fresh flavors and contrasting textures."

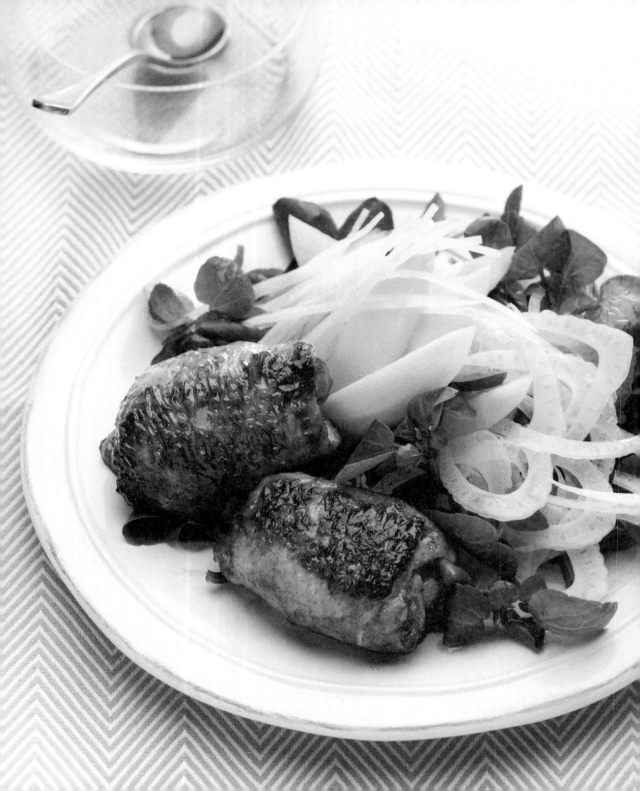

Ginger & Umeboshi Chicken

Umeboshi paste is a traditional Japanese condiment that has a fruity, sour and tangy flavor. It is combined here with ginger and honey to create a sticky glaze for chicken. The dish is served with a digestion-supporting salad of watercress, fennel and white radish.

1 Put the chicken in a shallow dish. Mix together the honey, umeboshi paste and spices. Pour the mixture over the chicken and leave to marinate 15 minutes.

2 Heat the olive oil in a skillet over medium heat, add the chicken thighs and cook 3 to 4 minutes until brown all over. Pour in the remaining marinade and the chicken stock. Cover the pan and simmer 6 to 7 minutes until the thighs are cooked through.

3 Toss the watercress, mango, daikon, fennel, lemon juice and oil lightly together in a bowl (or arrange the salad on plates and drizzle with the lemon and oil). Top with the chicken to serve. (Leftovers can be stored in the refrigerator up to 2 days.)

SERVES 4

PREPARATION TIME 10 minutes, plus 15 minutes marinating

COOKING TIME 10 minutes

8 boneless chicken thighs, with skin
3 tablespoons raw honey
1 tablespoon umeboshi paste/plum paste
¼-inch piece fresh gingerroot, peeled and grated
½ teaspoon Chinese five-spice powder
a pinch paprika
1 tablespoon olive oil or coconut oil
4 tablespoons chicken or vegetable stock
2 ounces watercress
1 small ripe mango, peeled, seeded and sliced
1 cup daikon or white radish, or kohlrabi, in matchstick strips
1 fennel bulb, thinly sliced
1 tablespoon lemon juice
1 tablespoon olive oil or flaxseed oil

NUTRITIONAL INFORMATION PER SERVING
Protein 27.3g, **Carbohydrates** 19.6g of which sugars 19.6g, **Fat** 15g of which saturates 4.8g, **Calories** 324

HEALTH BENEFITS
Umeboshi, made from Japanese pickled plum, is traditionally used in Japanese dishes to stimulate the digestion. The plums are also known for their health-giving alkalizing properties—an alkaline environment is thought to reduce the risk of cancer.

Turkey & Pistachio Korma

SERVES 4

PREPARATION TIME 15 minutes,
plus 30 minutes marinating

COOKING TIME 30 minutes

14 ounces boneless, skinless turkey
breast, sliced

3 tablespoons Greek or soy yogurt

½ teaspoon garam masala

¼-inch piece fresh gingerroot, grated

½ green chili, seeded and finely chopped
(optional)

½ teaspoon turmeric

1 teaspoon tamarind paste

1 garlic clove, crushed

Nut sauce

2 onions, finely chopped

½-inch piece fresh gingerroot, grated

½ teaspoon turmeric

2 garlic cloves, crushed

½ cup pistachios

1 tablespoon olive oil or coconut oil

scant 1 cup chicken stock

⅔ cup Greek or soy yogurt

7 ounces baby spinach leaves

2 tablespoons chopped cilantro leaves,
plus extra leaves to serve

Pistachios create a rich sauce in this well-rounded curry.
The addition of the spiced yogurt marinade keeps the
turkey moist and tender, and tamarind gives it a tangy
edge. For a dairy-free option you can use soy or coconut
yogurt instead of the Greek yogurt. Serve with steamed
vegetables and a little brown rice.

1 Put the turkey in a shallow dish. Mix the remaining
   ingredients together and rub into the turkey. Leave
   to marinate 30 minutes.

2 To make the nut sauce, put the onions, spices and garlic
   into a blender or food processor and pulse to make a paste.
   Lightly toast the nuts in a dry skillet over medium heat
   1 minute, then set the nuts aside. Add the olive oil to the
   pan and heat. Add the turkey and marinade, and cook
   2 to 3 minutes to brown the turkey. Add the paste and
   stir 2 minutes, then pour in the stock. Bring to a boil and
   simmer 15 minutes, or until the turkey is cooked.

3 Put the nuts and yogurt into a blender or food processor
   and process until smooth. Add the yogurt sauce to the pan
   with the spinach and cilantro, bring to a boil and simmer
   5 minutes, or until the spinach wilts. Serve sprinkled
   with extra cilantro leaves. (Store in the refrigerator up
   to 3 days.)

NUTRITIONAL INFORMATION PER SERVING
Protein 33.2g, **Carbohydrates** 14.1g of which sugars 10.4g, **Fat** 12.4g of which saturates 4g, **Calories** 301

HEALTH BENEFITS
Turkey is an excellent source of protein, useful for supporting muscle mass and preventing cachexia (weight loss) in cancer patients.

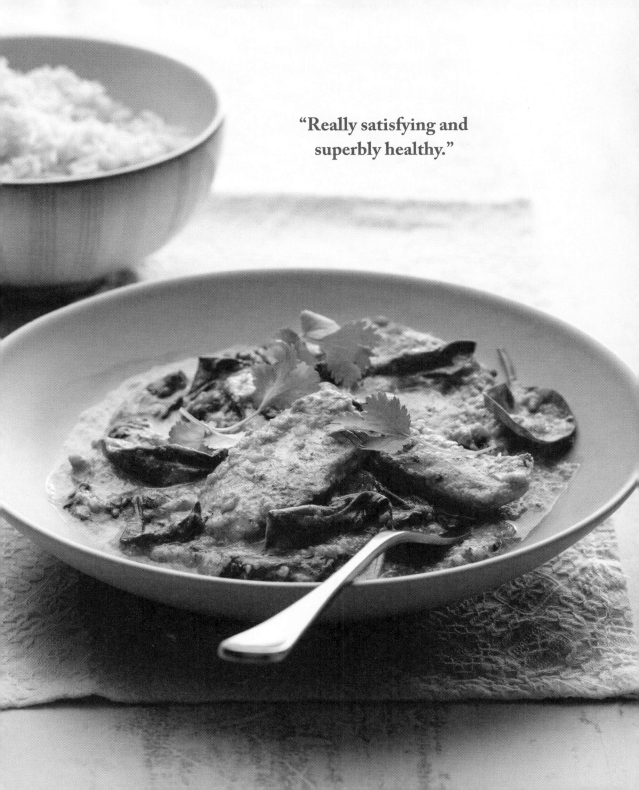

"Really satisfying and
superbly healthy."

Balsamic-Braised Duck

SERVES 4
PREPARATION TIME 15 minutes,
    plus 30 minutes marinating
COOKING TIME 20 minutes

4 boneless, skinless duck breast halves
1 tablespoon plus ⅔ cup balsamic vinegar
2 teaspoons raw honey
2 tablespoons tamari
1 cup dried shiitake mushrooms
1 tablespoon olive oil or coconut oil
2 onions, finely chopped
2 garlic cloves, crushed
3 cups sliced mixed mushrooms, including
    shiitake
1 cup plus 2 tablespoons chicken stock
1 tablespoon cornstarch
1 tablespoon cranberry or red currant jelly
1 handful parsley, leaves chopped
sea salt and freshly ground black pepper

Shiitake mushrooms add an intense flavor to this tangy sauce to accompany duck breasts. This attractive dish will tempt you to eat well when you may feel disinclined to prepare food. Serve with sweet potatoes and a salad.

1 Put the duck breasts into a shallow dish. Mix together the 1 tablespoon balsamic vinegar, the honey and tamari and pour it over the duck. Leave to marinate 30 minutes. Meanwhile, soak the mushrooms in boiling water to cover 15 minutes, then drain and reserve the liquid. Chop the mushrooms. Heat the oven to 375°F.

2 Heat an ovenproof skillet over medium heat and brown the duck on each side. Roast 12 to 15 minutes until cooked through. Leave to rest 5 minutes, then slice thinly.

3 Meanwhile, put the olive oil in the skillet and gently fry the onions and garlic 2 to 3 minutes until soft. Add all the mushrooms and stir 1 minute. Pour in the remaining vinegar, the stock and reserved mushroom liquid. Bring to a boil, then simmer 5 minutes. Mix the cornstarch with 2 tablespoons water, then add to the pan and stir until thick. Add the duck, cranberry jelly and parsley, then season and serve. (Store leftovers in the refrigerator up to 2 days.)

NUTRITIONAL INFORMATION PER SERVING
Protein 23.3g, **Carbohydrates** 14.4g of which sugars 7.1g, **Fat** 9.8g of which saturates 4.1g, **Calories** 246

HEALTH BENEFITS
Shiitake mushrooms have immune-boosting and cancer-protective properties, largely due to the presence of polysaccharides and polysaccharide glucans, which stimulate immune response and help macrophage cells in clearing potentially cancerous cells. They are also a source of vitamin D2, the B vitamins and the minerals manganese, phosphorus, potassium, selenium, copper and zinc.

Venison with Zesty Gremolata

Succulent and flavorsome venison is a good source
of protein, yet it is low in saturated fat. It benefits from
long, slow cooking, and here it is braised with vegetables
and olives to increase the depth of flavor. The orange
segments and gremolata contrast well with the richness of
the meat. Serve with steamed broccoli.

1 Heat the oven to 350°F. Heat 1 tablespoon of the olive
   oil in a Dutch oven over medium heat and gently fry the
   onion, celery, carrot and garlic 4 to 5 minutes until lightly
   colored. Remove from the pan and set aside.
2 Put the venison into a plastic bag with the flour and salt
   and pepper and shake to coat. Add a little more olive oil
   to the pan, if needed, then fry the venison in batches,
   stirring, until light brown all over.
3 Return the onion mixture to the pan, then add the wine,
   tomatoes, stock and olives. Bring to a boil, then cover and
   cook in the oven 1½ hours, or until tender.
4 Remove from the oven and check the seasoning. Stir in the
   orange segments. Mix together the zests with the parsley
   and scatter over the casserole. Serve. (Store leftovers in the
   refrigerator up to 2 days.)

SERVES 4
PREPARATION TIME 15 minutes
COOKING TIME 1 hour 45 minutes

1 to 2 tablespoons olive oil or coconut oil
1 onion, finely chopped
2 celery sticks, chopped
1 carrot, diced
2 garlic cloves, chopped
1 pound 5 ounces boneless venison
   shoulder or leg, cut into large chunks
3 tablespoons wholewheat flour
   or rice flour
1 cup plus 2 tablespoons red wine,
   or lamb or beef stock
1 can (15-oz.) crushed tomatoes
2 cups lamb or beef stock
1⅔ cups pitted green olives
2 oranges, in segments or thinly sliced
zest of 2 oranges
zest of 1 lemon
2 tablespoons finely chopped parsley
   leaves
sea salt and freshly ground black pepper

NUTRITIONAL INFORMATION PER SERVING
Protein 36.9g, **Carbohydrates** 18.5g of which sugars 9.7g, **Fat** 10.7g of which saturates 4.1g, **Calories** 361

HEALTH BENEFITS
Venison contains energizing iron and B vitamins, as well as zinc and selenium for immune and antioxidant support.

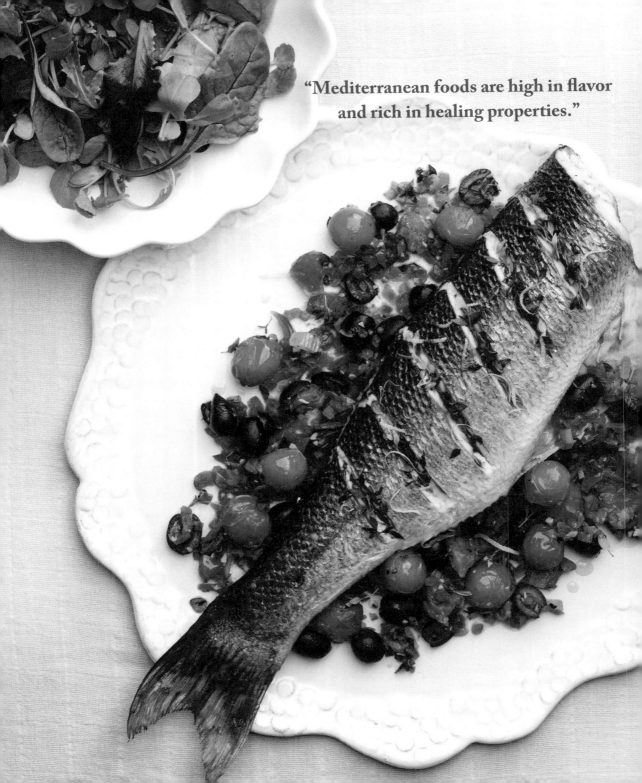

"Mediterranean foods are high in flavor and rich in healing properties."

Roasted Sea Bass with Olives & Tomatoes

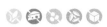

Roasting sea bass on a bed of Mediterranean vegetables makes it beautifully moist and full of flavor. This is simple to prepare, taking only 15 minutes, and is packed with antioxidant-rich and anti-inflammatory ingredients. Serve with salad, or steamed shredded kale or spinach.

1 Heat the oven to 375°F. Lightly toast the coriander seeds in a dry skillet over medium heat 1 minute, then crush using a mortar and pestle. Heat the olive oil in the skillet over medium heat. Add the onion, coriander and garlic and fry gently 2 to 3 minutes until the onion starts to become soft. Stir in the thyme leaves, olives and the sun-dried and cherry tomatoes.

2 Season with salt and pepper, then transfer to a large, shallow baking dish. Using a sharp knife, slash the skin of the fish diagonally on each side. Push sprigs of thyme into the cuts. Sprinkle the lemon zest over, then put the fish on top of the tomato mixture.

3 Drizzle a little olive oil over and roast 20 to 25 minutes until the fish is cooked through. Serve. (Store leftovers in the refrigerator up to 1 day.)

SERVES 4
PREPARATION TIME 15 minutes
COOKING TIME 30 minutes

½ teaspoon coriander seeds
1 tablespoon olive oil or coconut oil
1 red onion, roughly chopped
2 garlic cloves, crushed
leaves from 3 thyme sprigs, plus
   1 small bunch fresh thyme sprigs
1 cup pitted ripe olives, roughly chopped
½ cup drained and roughly chopped
   sun-dried tomatoes in oil
16 cherry tomatoes
1 large sea bass or trout, head removed,
   dressed
zest of 1 lemon
olive oil, for drizzling
sea salt and freshly ground black pepper

NUTRITIONAL INFORMATION PER SERVING
Protein 30.5g, **Carbohydrates** 3.4g of which sugars 2.7g, **Fat** 21.1g of which saturates 4.6g, **Calories** 323

HEALTH BENEFITS
Sea bass is a good source of omega-3 fats and also provides B vitamins, magnesium and the antioxidant mineral selenium.

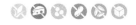

Salmon with Sauce Vierge

SERVES 4
PREPARATION TIME 10 minutes
COOKING TIME 10 minutes,
   plus 10 minutes infusing

½ cup, plus 1 tablespoon olive oil
zest and juice of 1 lemon
2 tomatoes, seeded and finely diced
1 shallot, finely chopped
2 garlic cloves, crushed
3 tablespoons chopped tarragon leaves
2 tablespoons chopped dill leaves
2 tablespoons chopped parsley leaves
2 tablespoons chopped chervil leaves
4 salmon fillets (about 5 ounces each),
   with skin
sea salt and freshly ground black pepper

A superbly healthy and flavorful dish. The light, herb sauce gives a fresh dimension to rich-tasting salmon. This dish is straightforward to prepare and can be made ahead and chilled until you are ready to cook. It's best to use wild salmon in preference to farmed. Serve with a salad of mixed leaves.

1 Pour the ½ cup olive oil into a small saucepan. Stir in the lemon zest and juice, then add the tomatoes, shallot and garlic. Heat the sauce very gently until just warm. Turn off the heat and add the herbs. Season with salt and pepper, then leave to infuse 10 minutes.

2 Season the salmon with black pepper to taste. Heat the 1 tablespoon olive oil in a skillet over medium heat. Add the salmon, skin side down, and fry 2 to 3 minutes until the skin is lightly colored.

3 Turn the fillets over and cook 2 to 3 minutes longer until the fish is cooked through. Pour the herb sauce into the skillet and warm through. Serve the salmon with the sauce spooned over.

NUTRITIONAL INFORMATION PER SERVING
Protein 23.3g, **Carbohydrates** 1.3g of which sugars 0.9g, **Fat** 46g of which saturates 8.6g, **Calories** 512

HEALTH BENEFITS
Salmon is high in protein and rich in omega-3 essential fatty acids. Fresh herbs contain antioxidants and volatile oils that possess cancer-protective properties.

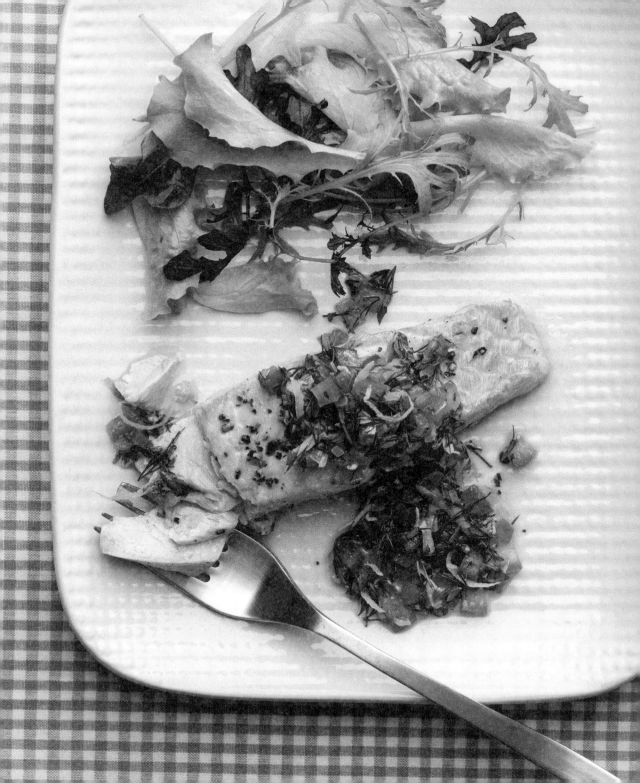

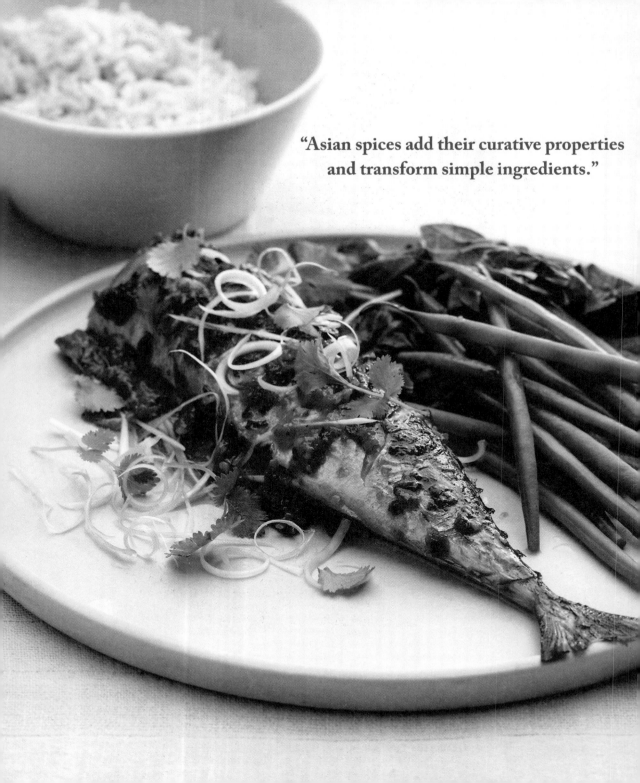

"Asian spices add their curative properties and transform simple ingredients."

Tamarind-Spiced Mackerel

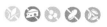

The rich, oily texture of mackerel contrasts well with the tangy, sour flavor of the tamarind in this Asian-inspired dish that is fragrant with lemongrass, ginger and mint. Oily fish is filling and sustaining, as well as being rich in omega-3 essential fats. Serve with brown rice, steamed spring or collard greens, green beans and scallions sprinkled over.

1 In a small bowl, mix together the tamarind, lemongrass, cayenne, if using, ginger, honey and mint.

2 Heat the broiler. Using a sharp knife, slash the skin of the mackerel on each side. Put the mackerel into a shallow flameproof dish and pour the tamarind sauce over. Coat thoroughly on both sides.

3 Put the dish under the broiler and broil 10 minutes, or until cooked through. Serve sprinkled with cilantro and scallions. (Leftovers can be stored in the refrigerator up to 1 day.)

SERVES 4
PREPARATION TIME 10 minutes
COOKING TIME 10 minutes

4 tablespoons tamarind paste
1 lemongrass stalk, tough parts removed, finely chopped
1 teaspoon cayenne pepper (optional)
½-inch piece fresh gingerroot, peeled and grated
2 tablespoons raw honey
1 small bunch mint, leaves chopped
4 mackerel, head removed and dressed
1 small handful cilantro leaves
2 scallions, finely sliced

NUTRITIONAL INFORMATION PER SERVING
Protein 38g, **Carbohydrates** 13.1g of which sugars 4.9g, **Fat** 32.4g of which saturates 6.6g, **Calories** 490

HEALTH BENEFITS
Tamarind is rich in soluble fiber, important for supporting bowel health and stabilizing blood sugar levels. It also contains antioxidants and phytochemicals, including limonene, known for its anticancer properties.

Miso-Glazed Salmon

SERVES 4

PREPARATION TIME 10 minutes,
 plus overnight marinating

COOKING TIME 25 minutes

1 pound 5 ounces salmon fillet, with skin,
 or 4 boneless salmon fillets (about
 5 ounces each), with skin

4 tablespoons Chinese rice wine

2 tablespoons mirin or 1 tablespoon rice
 wine

4 tablespoons white miso paste

1 tablespoon tamari

1 tablespoon xylitol or a pinch stevia
 (optional)

1 handful cilantro leaves, chopped

1 to 2 tablespoons lemon juice

Sweet and tangy miso is a nutritious ingredient that marries beautifully with omega-3-rich salmon fillets. Leaving the fish to marinate overnight guarantees it has plenty of flavor and will be moist and tender. Opt for wild salmon, if possible, because it has a higher proportion of omega-3 fats. Serve with stir-fried vegetables.

1 Put the salmon in a shallow, ceramic or glass baking dish. Mix together the remaining ingredients, except the cilantro and lemon juice, then pour over the fish to coat thoroughly. Cover with plastic wrap and leave to marinate in the refrigerator overnight.

2 Heat the oven to 400°F. Remove the plastic wrap, cover the dish with foil and put into the oven. Roast 15 minutes. Remove the foil and roast 5 to 10 minutes longer until the fish is cooked through. Scatter the cilantro leaves over and drizzle with lemon juice to taste before serving. (Store in the refrigerator up to 2 days.)

NUTRITIONAL INFORMATION PER SERVING
Protein 32.5g, **Carbohydrates** 7.1g of which sugars 3.6g, **Fat** 17.4g of which saturates 2.9g, **Calories** 324

HEALTH BENEFITS
Miso provides a good source of protective phytonutrients and antioxidants, including zinc and manganese.

Mixed Seafood Pie

Try this traditional fish pie with a healthy difference: the seafood mixture is topped with antioxidant-rich mashed sweet potatoes enriched with tahini. For a dairy-free pie, use soy, coconut or oat milk and cream. Serve with a crisp leafy green salad or lightly steamed broccoli and carrots.

1 Heat the oven to 350°F. To make the topping, boil the sweet potatoes 10 to 15 minutes until tender. Drain and set aside. Meanwhile, heat 1 tablespoon of the olive oil in a large skillet over medium heat. Add the onion and leek and gently fry 5 minutes. Add the fish to the pan and gently fry 1 to 2 minutes to seal.

2 Heat the remaining olive oil in a saucepan over medium heat. Stir in the flour and cook 1 minute. Remove the pan from the heat and gradually beat in the milk and cream. Return to the heat and bring to a boil, whisking constantly. Add the mustard, dill and nutmeg, then season.

3 Stir the fish, vegetables and shrimp into the sauce, then spoon into a baking dish. Mash the sweet potatoes and beat in the cream and tahini, then season. Spoon the mashed potatoes over the fish. Bake 20 to 30 minutes until golden. Serve. (Store leftovers in the refrigerator up to 2 days or freeze, uncooked, 1 month.)

SERVES 4

PREPARATION TIME 15 minutes

COOKING TIME 45 minutes

2 tablespoons olive oil or coconut oil

1 onion, finely chopped

1 leek, thinly sliced

7 ounces salmon fillet, skinned and cut into cubes

7 ounces white fish fillet, such as coley or haddock, skinned and cut into cubes

¼ cup all-purpose flour

1¾ cups 2% milk or dairy-free milk

2 tablespoons light cream, or oat or soy cream

4 teaspoons wholegrain mustard

1 handful dill leaves, chopped

a pinch freshly grated nutmeg

5 ounces shelled cooked shrimp

sea salt and freshly ground black pepper

Sweet potato topping

4 cups sweet potato chunks

2 tablespoons light cream, or oat or soy cream

1 tablespoon tahini

NUTRITIONAL INFORMATION PER SERVING

Protein 34.6g, **Carbohydrates** 37.3g of which sugars 10.5g, **Fat** 18.3g of which saturates 7.6g, **Calories** 454

HEALTH BENEFITS

Sweet potatoes are rich in antioxidants, especially carotenoids and vitamins A and C.

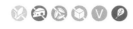

Roasted Tempeh with Pipérade Sauce

SERVES 4
PREPARATION TIME 15 minutes
COOKING TIME 30 minutes

2 tablespoons olive oil or coconut oil
2 red onions, sliced
6 garlic cloves, chopped
2 cups drained and chopped roasted red
  bell peppers from a jar
4 vine-ripened tomatoes, roughly
  chopped
1 tablespoon sun-dried tomato paste
a pinch smoked or sweet paprika
3 tablespoons apple cider vinegar
  or sherry vinegar
1 pound tempeh, cut into ¾-inch cubes
olive oil, for drizzling
3 tablespoons roughly chopped parsley
  leaves (optional)
sea salt and freshly ground black pepper

Bell peppers, garlic, tomatoes and onions form the base of the pipérade. If you can find sherry vinegar, its flavor and potent antioxidant and anti-inflammatory qualities add to the dish. The tempeh readily absorbs the rich flavors of this sauce while it's cooking. Serve with salad.

1 Heat the oven to 375°F. Heat a skillet over medium heat and add 1 tablespoon of the olive oil. Fry the onions 2 minutes, or until just soft. Add the garlic, peppers, tomatoes, sun-dried tomato paste and paprika and continue cooking over low heat 5 minutes, or until soft.

2 Put the mixture into a food processor and pulse briefly until coarsely chopped—it should still be chunky. Stir in the vinegar.

3 Heat the remaining oil in the skillet and add the tempeh. Fry 10 to 12 minutes until golden. Tip the tempeh into a baking dish and pour the sauce over. Drizzle a little olive oil over and roast 15 minutes, or until the sauce is thick and bubbling. Stir in the parsley, if using, season and serve. (Store in the refrigerator up to 2 days.)

NUTRITIONAL INFORMATION PER SERVING
Protein 25.4g, **Carbohydrates** 16.7g of which sugars 9.9g, **Fat** 13.1g of which saturates 4.2g, **Calories** 291

HEALTH BENEFITS
Tempeh is a highly nutritious fermented food made from soybeans, with a high protein content. It has been a staple in Indonesia for more than 2,000 years. Tempeh is rich in essential fatty acids and numerous vitamins, minerals and health-promoting isoflavones.

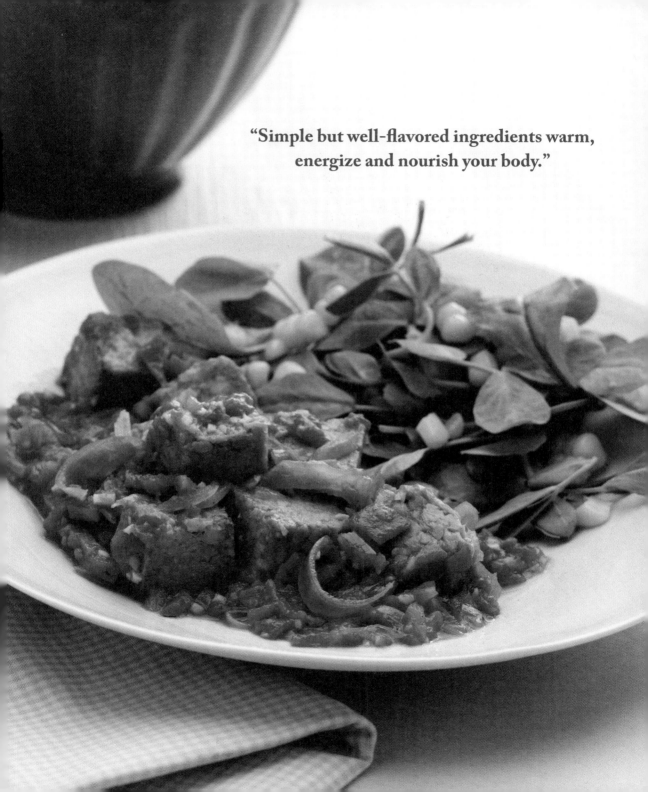

"Simple but well-flavored ingredients warm, energize and nourish your body."

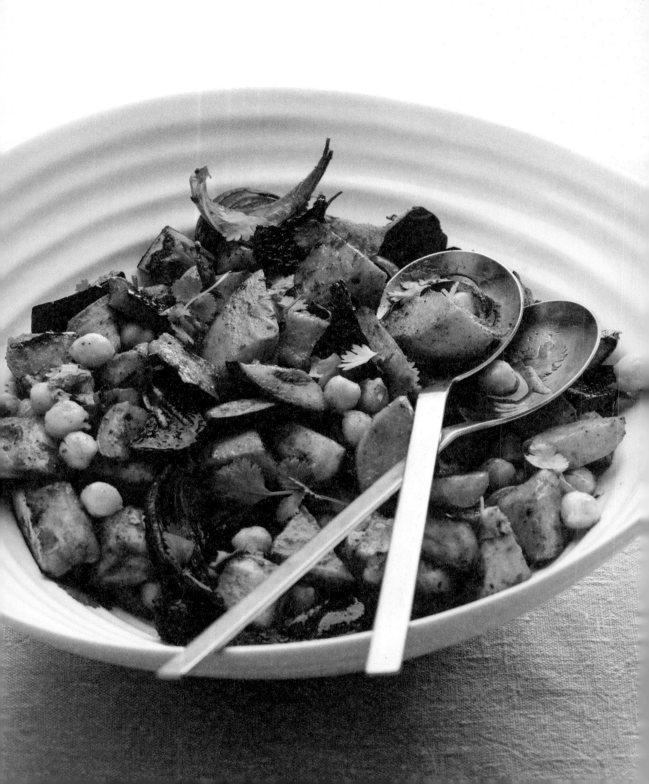

Warm Eggplant, Roots & Chickpea Salad

Cumin and paprika make a tangy, spicy dressing to add to this robust, warm salad of roasted vegetables and chickpeas. If you prefer a little extra protein, you can also serve it with hard-boiled egg, tofu or feta cheese—or, for nonvegetarians, serve with cooked chicken.

1 Heat the oven to 400°F. Put the onion, sweet potato, carrots and beets into a baking dish. Mix together the oil, spices, garlic, lemon zest and juice. Pour this mixture over the vegetables and toss to coat.

2 Put in the oven and roast 15 minutes. Add the eggplants to the dish and toss to coat in the oil. Bake 15 minutes longer, or until the vegetables are tender and lightly colored. Remove the dish from the oven. Tip the chickpeas into the dish with the cilantro.

3 Mix together the dressing ingredients. Drizzle the dressing over the vegetables to serve. (Store in the refrigerator up to 2 days.)

SERVES 4
PREPARATION TIME 10 minutes
COOKING TIME 30 minutes

1 red onion, cut into wedges
1 sweet potato, cut into chunks
2 carrots, cut into large chunks
2 small beets, cut into wedges
2 tablespoons olive oil or melted
    coconut oil
1 teaspoon each paprika and
    ground cumin
1 garlic clove, crushed
zest and juice of ½ lemon
2 eggplants, cut into chunks
1 can (15-oz.) chickpeas, drained
    and rinsed
3 tablespoons chopped cilantro leaves

Spicy dressing
½ teaspoon ground cumin
a pinch paprika
2 teaspoons raw honey or manuka honey
juice of 1 lemon
4 tablespoons olive oil or flaxseed oil

NUTRITIONAL INFORMATION PER SERVING
Protein 7.2g, **Carbohydrates** 31.7g of which sugars 15.2g, **Fat** 16.1g of which saturates 5.5g, **Calories** 298

HEALTH BENEFITS
Eggplants, beets and other purple-colored fruit and vegetables contain anthocyanins, which have been shown to attack cancer cells. Chickpeas, like other beans and legumes, are a good source of phytoestrogens (plant estrogens), shown to protect against the spread of hormonally driven cancers.

Spaghetti with Lemon & Broccoli

SERVES 4
PREPARATION TIME 10 minutes
COOKING TIME 10 minutes

10 ounces wholewheat or spelt spaghetti
2¼ pounds broccoli, cut into small florets
1 tablespoon olive oil or coconut oil
2 garlic cloves, crushed
2 red chilies, seeded and finely chopped
  (optional)
4 scallions, thinly sliced
zest of 1 lemon
1½ cups crumbled feta cheese
juice of ½ lemon
freshly ground black pepper

A simple, fast dish containing broccoli, garlic, chili and onions—all of which are beneficial for the recovery from cancer. The addition of feta cheese provides protein, but for a dairy-free option, add cooked chicken breast or drained and rinsed canned mixed beans.

1 Cook the pasta in boiling water 7 to 8 minutes until tender but with a little bite, or according to the package directions. Drain.

2 Meanwhile, put the broccoli in a steamer and steam over high heat 3 minutes, or until just tender. Set aside.

3 Heat a skillet over medium heat and add the olive oil. Gently fry the garlic, chilies, if using, scallions and lemon zest 2 to 3 minutes until the scallions are just soft. Add the broccoli and heat through. Tip the broccoli mixture into the pasta with the feta cheese and lemon juice and toss well. Season with black pepper, then serve. (Store in the refrigerator up to 1 day.)

NUTRITIONAL INFORMATION PER SERVING
Protein 29.1g, **Carbohydrates** 51.6g of which sugars 7.3g, **Fat** 16.5g of which saturates 9.6g, **Calories** 474

HEALTH BENEFITS
Both wholewheat and spelt spaghetti have a lower glycemic index than white pasta, meaning the effect on blood sugar levels is reduced, and they also provide a useful source of dietary fiber.

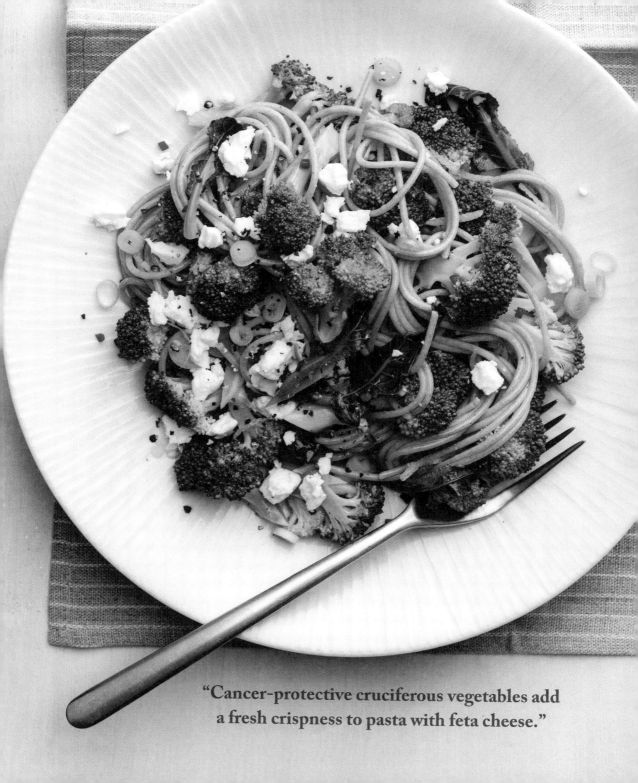

"Cancer-protective cruciferous vegetables add a fresh crispness to pasta with feta cheese."

Hempseed & Nut Burgers

SERVES 4
PREPARATION TIME 10 minutes,
    plus 30 minutes chilling
COOKING TIME 40 minutes

1 tablespoon olive oil or coconut oil
1 red onion, finely chopped
1 carrot, grated
1¼ cups finely chopped mushrooms
1 garlic clove, crushed
¾ cup drained and rinsed canned
    cannellini beans
scant ½ cup walnut pieces
⅓ cup cashews
2 tablespoons shelled hempseed
1 cup fresh wholewheat bread crumbs,
    or gluten-free bread crumbs
    or rolled oats
1 tablespoon tamari
2 teaspoons raw honey
1 egg yolk
sea salt and freshly ground black pepper

Homemade vegetarian burgers taste wholesome and satisfying. Full of fiber, protein and healthy fats, these hempseed and nut burgers make a popular family meal, and because they can be frozen, they are useful to make ahead for those days when a quickly cooked meal is all you want. Serve with a salad and a salsa or Celery Root, Apple & Fennel Rémoulade (page 88).

1 Heat the olive oil in a large skillet over medium heat and add the onion, carrot, mushrooms and garlic. Gently fry 10 minutes, or until the vegetables are soft and the liquid evaporates. Add the beans to the pan and cook 1 minute longer. Leave the mixture to cool slightly.
2 Put the nuts in a food processor and pulse until coarsely chopped. Add the bean mixture and the remaining ingredients and pulse again to combine. Chill 30 minutes. Heat the oven to 375°F and line a baking tray with baking parchment.
3 Shape the mixture into 8 burgers. Put onto the baking tray and bake 20 to 30 minutes until crisp and lightly colored. Serve. (Store in the refrigerator up to 3 days or freeze, uncooked, up to 3 months.)

NUTRITIONAL INFORMATION PER SERVING
Protein 5.9g, **Carbohydrates** 11.4g of which sugars 3.3g, **Fat** 11.1g of which saturates 1.6g, **Calories** 169

HEALTH BENEFITS
Using hempseed and nuts in these burgers increases their protein content and provides essential omega-3 and -6 fats. Walnuts are also rich in antioxidant phenols and vitamin E. They are a valuable anticancer food and their consumption has been shown to reduce the risk of certain cancers, including prostate and breast cancer.

Persian Quinoa Omega Bowl

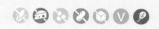

This versatile Middle Eastern-inspired salad is packed with colorful vegetables, grains and legumes, pomegranate seeds and berries, plus omega-rich seeds and oils. Add a poached egg or feta cheese if you want more protein. Any leftovers make a good packed lunch.

1 Heat the oven to 350°F. Put the eggplant, pepper and squash into a baking dish and toss with the 3 tablespoons olive oil and the cumin. Season with salt and pepper and roast 30 minutes, or until tender.

2 Meanwhile, put the quinoa into a saucepan with 1½ cups water and the saffron, if using. Bring to a boil, cover and reduce the heat to a very low simmer. Simmer 15 minutes, then turn off the heat and keep covered 5 minutes longer.

3 Meanwhile, put the green beans in a steamer and steam over high heat 2 minutes. Drain and refresh under cold water. Tip the quinoa into a large bowl and add the cooked vegetables, lentils, seeds, berries and tomatoes.

4 Mix together the olive oil, the lemon zest and juice and mint. Pour it over the salad and toss to coat before serving. (Store in the refrigerator up to 3 days.)

SERVES 6
PREPARATION TIME 15 minutes
COOKING TIME 30 minutes

1 small eggplant, cut into ¾-inch chunks
1 red bell pepper, seeded and cut into chunks
1½ cups diced butternut squash
3 tablespoons olive oil
1 teaspoon cumin seeds
scant 1 cup quinoa
½ teaspoon saffron threads (optional)
⅔ cup green beans cut in half
1 can (15-oz.) Puy lentils, drained and rinsed
6 tablespoons mixed seeds, such as pumpkin, sunflower and shelled hempseed
3 tablespoons pomegranate seeds
3 tablespoons dried unsweetened berries
8 cherry tomatoes, cut in half
4 tablespoons olive oil or flaxseed oil
zest and juice of 1 lemon
3 tablespoons chopped mint leaves
sea salt and freshly ground black pepper

NUTRITIONAL INFORMATION PER SERVING
Protein 14.6g, **Carbohydrates** 33.5g of which sugars 13g, **Fat** 27.1g of which saturates 3g, **Calories** 442

HEALTH BENEFITS
Quinoa is a nutritious, gluten-free grainlike seed that is high in protein, containing all nine essential amino acids. It contains magnesium for energy production and is a source of manganese, which helps to protect cells from oxidative damage.

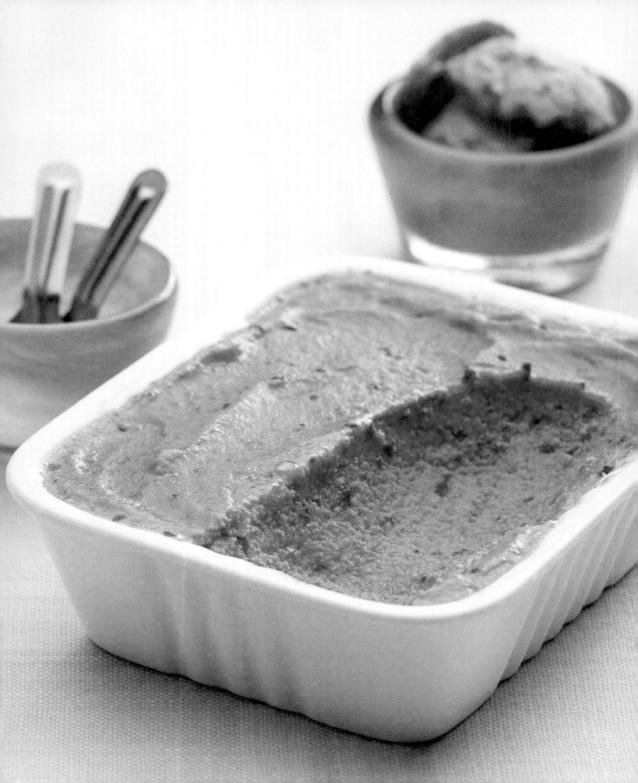

Desserts &
Baked Treats

Cancer treatments can often increase the cravings for something sweet,
especially for patients who experience a bitter or metallic taste in their mouths.
In this chapter you will find a range of low-sugar recipes for desserts, as well
as baked treats—perfect for when you are traveling and for packed lunches.
None contain refined sugar and all are carefully balanced to help stabilize
blood sugar. Rather than providing empty calories,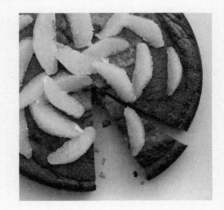
these dishes are rich with nutritious ingredients and
designed to support energy levels. There is a range
of tempting desserts, including Apple, Walnut &
Pistachio Crumble and Gooey Chocolate & Raspberry
Pudding. Among the cakes and baked treats are
Matcha Tea & Banana Bread or, for a savory option,
Savory Onion & Kale Chips and Spiced Flatbreads.

Opposite: Super-Berry Yogurt Sorbet (page 126)
Above: Almond-Citrus Cake (page 125)

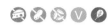

Gooey Chocolate & Raspberry Pudding

SERVES 4
PREPARATION TIME 10 minutes
COOKING TIME 40 minutes

oil, for greasing
1 cup wholewheat flour or gluten-free
    flour mix
2 teaspoons baking powder
1 tablespoon unsweetened cocoa powder
1 teaspoon vanilla extract
½ cup sugar-free apple puree
½ cup soy milk
1 tablespoon xylitol
1¼ cups raspberries, plus extra to serve
    (optional)

Chocolate sauce
2 tablespoons xylitol
1 heaped tablespoon unsweetened
    cocoa powder

Beneath a light chocolate cake studded with fresh raspberries lies an intense chocolate sauce. Perhaps surprisingly, this is a healthy dish, because it uses pureed apple and xylitol to give it a touch of sweetness.

1 Heat the oven to 350°F and lightly grease a round 8-inch baking dish. Sift the flour, baking powder and cocoa powder into a bowl, then tip in the bran left in the sifter.

2 Mix together the vanilla, apple puree, milk and xylitol and beat into the flour mixture. Stir in the raspberries, then spoon into the baking dish.

3 Combine the sauce ingredients with 1¾ cups boiling water, and pour gently over the batter. Do not stir the liquid in— it will seep in as the pudding bakes.

4 Carefully put the dish in the oven and leave to bake 35 to 40 minutes until the pudding is firm on top but with a gooey chocolate sauce underneath. Serve with extra raspberries, if you like. (Store leftovers in the refrigerator up to 2 days.)

NUTRITIONAL INFORMATION PER SERVING
Protein 5.4g, **Carbohydrates** 38.7g of which sugars 14.8g, **Fat** 2.2g of which of saturates 0.8g, **Calories** 181

HEALTH BENEFITS
Polyphenols, in the cocoa powder, are known for their antioxidant properties. For a stronger antioxidant boost you can use high-antioxidant cocoa powder, available from health food stores and online suppliers. It has a slightly stronger, bitter taste, so use a little less in the recipe and increase the amount of xylitol slightly.

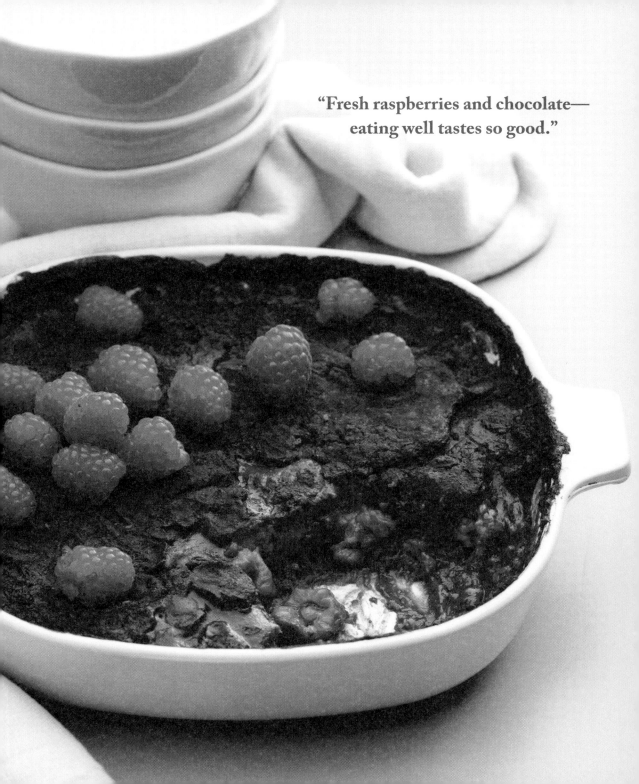

"Fresh raspberries and chocolate—
eating well tastes so good."

2 tablespoons olive oil or coconut oil, plus
   extra for greasing
3 pounds cooking apples, peeled and cut
   into chunks
1 teaspoon cinnamon
3 tablespoons xylitol
1 tablespoon apple concentrate or raw
   honey

Crumble topping
¾ cup unsweetened shredded coconut
scant 1 cup pistachios
1 cup walnut pieces
a pinch sea salt
¾ cup rolled oats or buckwheat flakes
3 small pitted dried dates

Apple, Walnut & Pistachio Crumble

Try this healthy version of the warming crumble with a topping of ground nuts and oats sweetened with dates. You don't have to bake the crumble topping—you can simply sprinkle it over the cooked apples and serve, if you prefer. Plain yogurt goes very well with this.

1 Heat the oven to 400°F and grease a baking dish. Heat a saucepan over medium heat and add the olive oil, apples, cinnamon, xylitol and apple concentrate, then cook 5 to 8 minutes until the apples are soft. Add a splash of water, if necessary, to prevent the mixture drying out. Transfer the apples to the dish.

2 To make the crumble, put the coconut, nuts and salt into a food processor and process to form crumbs. Pulse in the oats and dates to form coarse crumbs. Sprinkle the topping over the apples, then bake 15 to 20 minutes until golden and bubbling. Serve hot or warm. (Leftovers can be stored in the refrigerator up to 2 days.)

NUTRITIONAL INFORMATION PER SERVING
Protein 6.8g, **Carbohydrates** 32.1g of which sugars 27.3g, **Fat** 24.4g of which saturates 7.2g, **Calories** 368

HEALTH BENEFITS
Apples are rich in polyphenols—antioxidants shown to help balance blood sugar levels and reduce glucose spikes. They also provide soluble fiber, including pectin, which has been shown to help with the excretion of fat and cholesterol from the body.

Baked Lemon Cheesecake

This is a creamy, dairy-free cheesecake low in sugar, but high in protein and isoflavones. A little xylitol and some dates provide sweetness, and the cheesecake is served with an antioxidant-rich berry sauce. Behind its indulgent appearance and taste is a healthy dessert that's perfect for entertaining, too.

1 Heat the oven to 350°F and lightly grease an 8-inch springform cake pan. Put the oat crackers and coconut into a food processor and pulse to form fine crumbs. Add the butter, dates, lemon zest and juice. Process to form a sticky dough. Spoon into the pan and press onto the bottom.

2 Put the filling ingredients into the food processor and process until smooth. Pour over the crumb crust, then bake 35 to 40 minutes until firm. Turn off the oven and leave the cheesecake to cool in the oven 30 minutes.

3 Meanwhile, to make the sauce, mix the cornstarch with 2 tablespoons water. Put the berries into a saucepan with the cornstarch mixture and simmer 1 to 2 minutes, stirring, until thick. Leave to cool. Serve the cheesecake with the sauce. (Store leftovers in the refrigerator up to 4 days.)

SERVES 8

PREPARATION TIME 15 minutes

COOKING TIME 45 minutes, plus cooling

¼ cup butter, melted, or melted coconut oil, plus extra for greasing

5 ounces oat crackers, rough oatcakes or gluten-free oatcakes

heaped 1 cup unsweetened shredded coconut

3 small pitted dried dates

zest and juice of 1 lemon

Tofu filling

1 pound 2 ounces silken tofu or firm tofu

zest of 4 lemons and juice of 1

⅓ cup xylitol

3 egg yolks

¼ cup cornstarch

Berry sauce

1 tablespoon cornstarch

2 cups fresh or frozen mixed berries

NUTRITIONAL INFORMATION PER SERVING
Protein 9.4g, **Carbohydrates** 33.1g of which sugars 15.8g, **Fat** 22.1g of which saturates 14.4g, **Calories** 359

HEALTH BENEFITS
The tofu and eggs are protein rich and low in sugar. Berries are a good source of phytonutrients, including cancer-protective chemicals, such as ellagic acid (richest in strawberries and raspberries) and anthocyanosides (richest in blueberries).

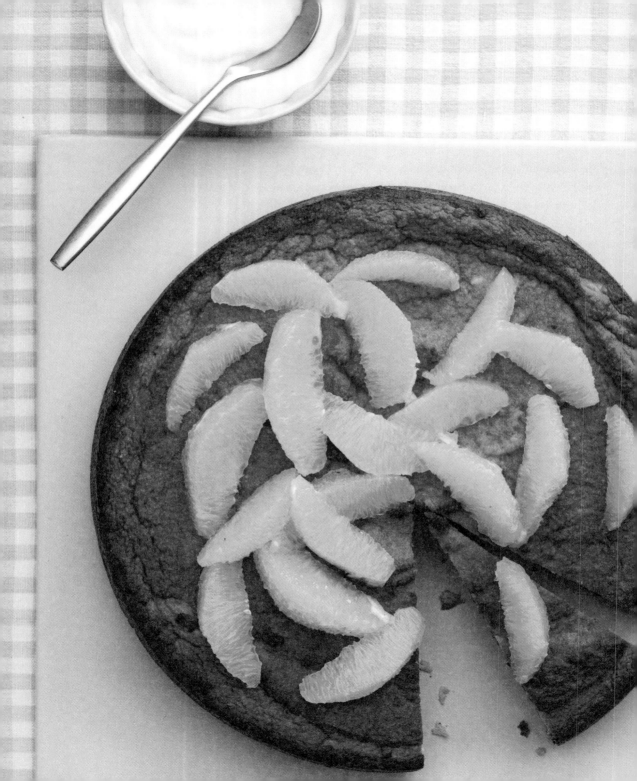

Almond-Citrus Cake

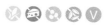

The oranges in this moist dessert cake give it a vibrant tang. It can be served warm or cold accompanied with soy or plain yogurt and orange segments or any other fresh fruit. Using olive oil, rich in omega-9, is an easy way to cram healthy anti-inflammatory fats into your diet, and using ground almonds instead of all-purpose flour keeps this cake gluten-free and high in protein.

1 Boil the oranges whole 1½ hours, or until soft. Heat the oven to 350°F and grease a round 9-inch cake pan.

2 Put the whole oranges into a blender or food processor and process until smooth. Add the lemon zest, eggs, xylitol, oil, almonds, salt and baking soda, then pulse until thoroughly mixed. Pour the batter into the prepared cake pan.

3 Bake 45 to 50 minutes until a skewer inserted into the middle comes out clean. Leave the cake to cool in the pan on a wire rack before turning out. Serve with fresh fruit, if you like. (Store, wrapped, in the refrigerator up to 3 days or freeze up to 3 months.)

SERVES 12

PREPARATION TIME 10 minutes

COOKING TIME 2 hours 20 minutes, plus cooling

2 oranges, washed
3 tablespoons olive oil, plus extra for greasing
zest of 1 lemon
4 eggs
⅓ cup xylitol
2½ cups very finely ground blanched almonds
½ teaspoon sea salt
1 teaspoon baking soda
fresh fruit, to serve (optional)

NUTRITIONAL INFORMATION PER SERVING
Protein 6.7g, **Carbohydrates** 7.9g of which sugars 7.2g, **Fat** 15.8g of which saturates 1.8g, **Calories** 193

HEALTH BENEFITS
Using the whole oranges, including the peel, retains the citrus flavanones, which tend to be concentrated around the pith and peel. These phytonutrients have been shown to be particularly powerful against many types of cancers.

Green Tea Ice Cream

SERVES 6
PREPARATION TIME 10 minutes,
  plus 2 hours freezing

¾ cup cashews
¼ cup plain or vanilla protein powder
  (such as whey or rice) (optional)
¾ cup plus 2 tablespoons coconut water
  or water
1 tablespoon raw honey (optional)
3 mint leaves
1 teaspoon matcha green tea powder
4 bananas, sliced and frozen

1 Put all the ingredients, except the bananas, into a blender or food processor. Process until smooth. Add the bananas and process. Serve at once or freeze. (Store in the freezer up to 3 months; allow to soften slightly before serving.)

NUTRITIONAL INFORMATION PER SERVING
Protein 6.8g, **Carbohydrates** 23.7g of which sugars 17.9g,
Fat 10.1g of which saturates 2g, **Calories** 214

HEALTH BENEFITS
Matcha is exceptionally high in antioxidants and contains a potent class of antioxidant known as catechins. Green tea is also rich in L-theanine, an amino acid that promotes a state of relaxation and well-being by creating alpha waves in the brain.

Super-Berry Yogurt Sorbet ▶

SERVES 4
PREPARATION TIME: 5 minutes,
  plus 3 hours freezing

¾ cup plus 2 tablespoons plain yogurt,
  soy yogurt or coconut yogurt
2 teaspoons acai berry powder (optional)
scant 1 cup strawberries
1 cup raspberries
1½ cups fresh or frozen pitted cherries

1 Put all the ingredients into a blender or food processor and process until smooth. Pour into a shallow freezerproof container and freeze 2 to 3 hours until firm. Remove from the freezer 30 minutes before serving to soften slightly. (Store in the freezer up to 3 months.)

NUTRITIONAL INFORMATION PER SERVING
Protein 4g, **Carbohydrates** 12.2g of which sugars 11.5g,
Fat 5.3g of which saturates 3.4g, **Calories** 110

HEALTH BENEFITS
The probiotic plain yogurt supports your immune system and digestive health. The optional acai berry powder provides additional antioxidant benefits.

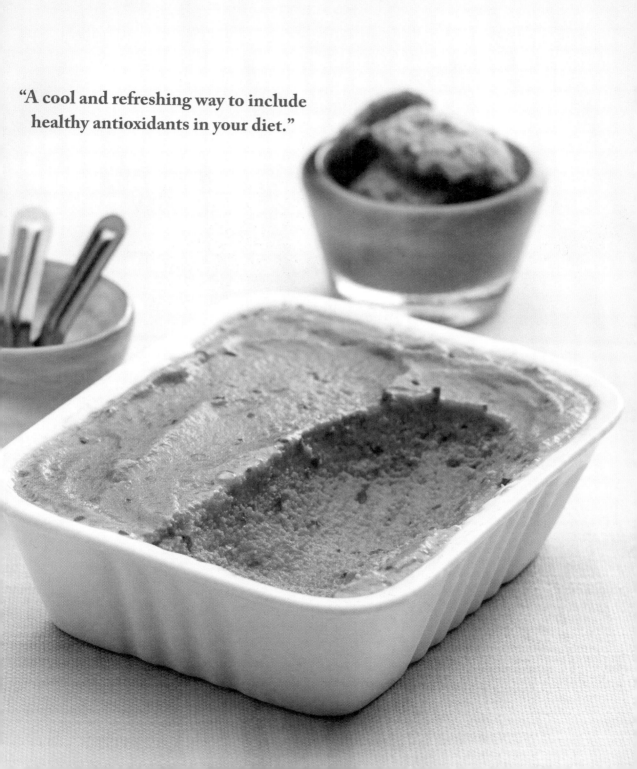

"A cool and refreshing way to include healthy antioxidants in your diet."

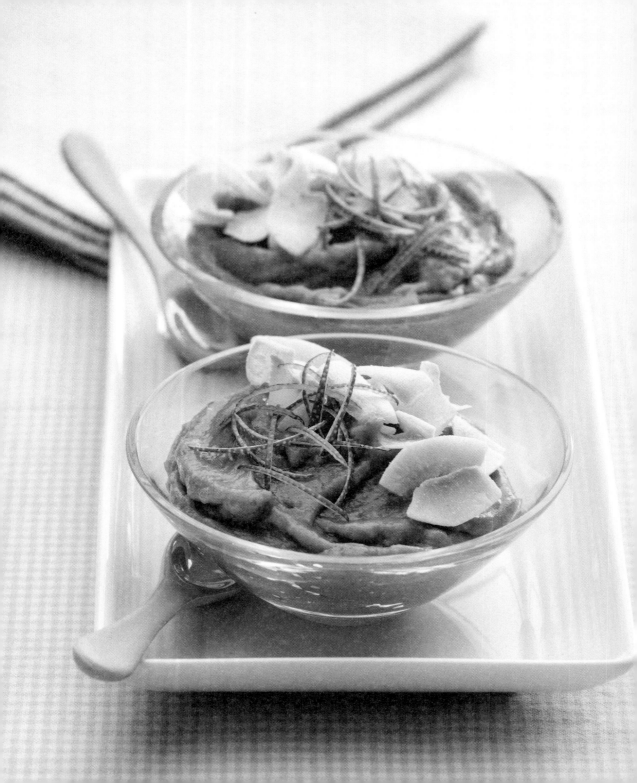

Avocado & Lime Mousse

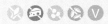

Tangy, zesty and refreshing, this simple dessert combines lime juice with creamy avocado and sweet dates to create a sensational, but healthy, mousse. Qualities include good fats, vitamins E and C, beta-carotenes and phytonutrients. The mousse can be prepared in advance and chilled until needed.

1 With a sharp knife, remove the zest in strips from the whole limes and remove any seeds. Reserve the zest. Put the limes and the remaining ingredients into a blender or food processor and process until smooth and creamy.

2 Spoon into 4 individual dishes and chill 1 to 2 hours before serving. Cut the zest into fine strips and use to decorate the mousses, then top with a sprinkling of coconut flakes before serving. (Store in the refrigerator up to 1 day.)

SERVES 4

PREPARATION TIME 5 minutes, plus 1 to 2 hours chilling

2 whole limes
juice of 2 limes
2 ripe avocados, seeded and peeled
5 pitted dried dates
1 tablespoon raw honey or manuka honey (optional)
2 tablespoons unsweetened coconut flakes, to serve

NUTRITIONAL INFORMATION PER SERVING
Protein 2.5g, **Carbohydrates** 21.4g of which sugars 21.2g, **Fat** 13g of which saturates 4.8g, **Calories** 213

HEALTH BENEFITS
Avocados contain B vitamins, including folic acid and B6. The optional manuka honey is well known for its antibacterial and antifungal properties and is useful for soothing sore throats, ulcers and wounds, as well as supporting energy levels and aiding digestion. The active ingredient found in manuka, but not present in other honeys, is known as UMF (unique manuka factor).

Matcha Tea & Banana Bread

MAKES 1 cake, 10 slices

PREPARATION TIME 15 minutes

COOKING TIME 45 minutes, plus
   cooling

½ cup unsalted butter, melted, or melted
   coconut oil, plus extra for greasing

1¼ cups wholewheat flour, or gluten-free
   flour mix plus ½ teaspoon xanthan gum

2 teaspoons matcha green tea powder,
   or 1 tablespoon ground green tea leaves

1 tablespoon baking powder

1 teaspoon cinnamon

3 tablespoons ground flaxseed

4 tablespoons unsweetened shredded
   coconut

⅔ cup ready-to-eat dried apricots,
   chopped

3 bananas, mashed

2 eggs

⅓ cup xylitol

An antioxidant-packed version of an all-time favorite, containing matcha—powdered green tea. This recipe is much lower in sugar than traditional quick breads, using fresh and dried fruit for sweetness.

1 Heat the oven to 350°F, then grease and line the bottom of an 8½- × 4½-inch bread pan with baking parchment. Sift the flour, matcha, baking powder and cinnamon into a bowl and tip in any bran remaining in the sifter. Stir in the flaxseed, 2 tablespoons of the coconut and the chopped apricots.

2 Pour the melted butter into a blender or food processor, add the bananas, eggs and xylitol and process until smooth. Add to the flour mixture and stir thoroughly. Spoon the mixture into the bread pan and sprinkle the remaining coconut over.

3 Bake 40 to 45 minutes until firm and lightly colored and a skewer inserted into the middle comes out clean. If the top begins to brown too much, cover with foil. Leave to cool in the pan 10 minutes, then turn out onto a wire rack to cool completely before serving. (Store, wrapped, in the refrigerator up to 3 days or freeze 1 month.)

NUTRITIONAL INFORMATION PER SLICE

Protein 5.8g, **Carbohydrates** 24.2g of which sugars 13.9g, **Fat** 15.1g of which saturates 8.4g, **Calories** 247

HEALTH BENEFITS

Eating matcha—the whole leaf of green tea—gives you the benefit of its plentiful antioxidants. Using wholewheat flour and ground flaxseed adds nutrients, including lignans, omega-3 fats and soluble fiber. The B vitamins, magnesium and selenium boost energy levels.

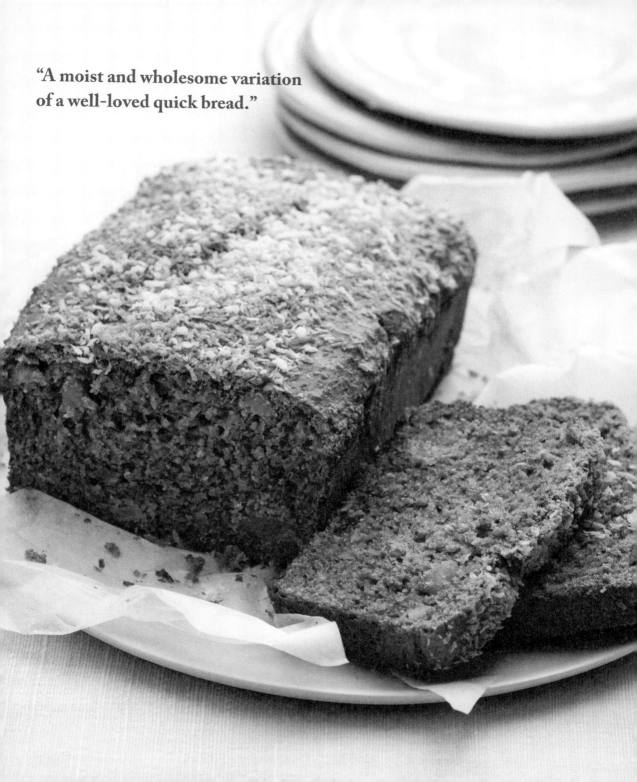

"A moist and wholesome variation of a well-loved quick bread."

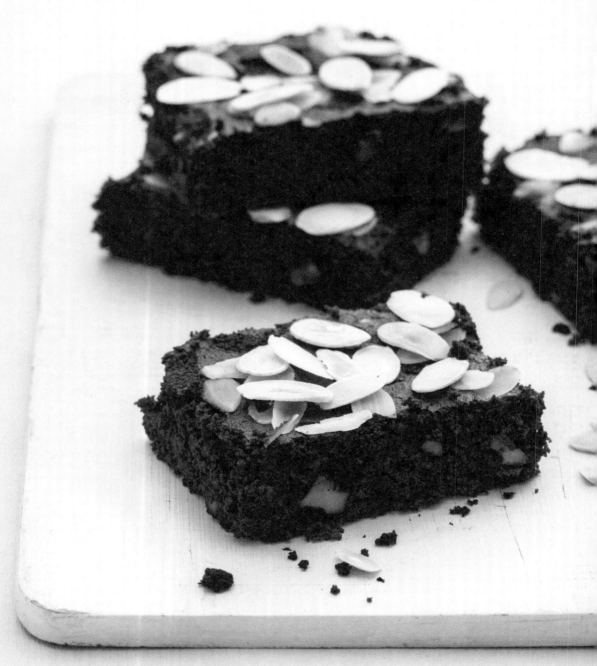

"The nourishing answer when you're feeling
tired and prefer to eat something sweet."

Chocolate & Beet Bars

MAKES 10
PREPARATION TIME 10 minutes
COOKING TIME 30 minutes,
   plus cooling

¼ cup butter or coconut oil, plus extra
   for greasing
9 ounces dairy-free dark chocolate
3 tablespoons xylitol
4 eggs
scant 1 cup roughly chopped cooked beet
1 cup very finely ground blanched
   almonds
a pinch sea salt
½ teaspoon cinnamon
½ teaspoon baking soda
½ cup walnut pieces, chopped
2 tablespoons slivered almonds

Similar to chocolate brownies, but much healthier, these bars are the perfect pick-me-up to restore flagging energy levels. A beet is added to the chocolate batter because of the soft and moist crumb it produces, and here it is combined with nuts for added flavor and texture.

1 Heat the oven to 350°F. Grease a shallow 12- × 8-inch baking pan and line with baking parchment. Put the chocolate, xylitol and butter into a saucepan and heat gently to melt the chocolate. Put the eggs and beet into a blender or food processor and process until smooth.

2 Tip the ground almonds into a large bowl. Add the melted chocolate mixture, the beet mixture and the remaining ingredients, except the slivered almonds. Mix well.

3 Pour the batter into the pan, then scatter the slivered almonds over. Bake 20 to 25 minutes until firm and the almonds are lightly colored. Leave to cool in the pan on a wire rack, then cut into bars to serve. (Store in an airtight container in the refrigerator up to 4 days or freeze 1 month.)

NUTRITIONAL INFORMATION PER BAR
Protein 7.7g, **Carbohydrates** 21.1g of which sugars 20.6g, **Fat** 26.6g of which saturates 11g, **Calories** 349

HEALTH BENEFITS
The almonds and walnuts increase the protein content, which helps to balance blood sugar. They also supply healthy fats, vitamins and minerals, including manganese, vitamin E, calcium and magnesium. Beets are rich in cancer-protective nutrients, including antioxidants, such as betalains, which have been shown to lessen tumor cell growth.

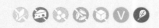

SERVES 8
PREPARATION TIME 10 minutes
COOKING TIME 20 minutes,
    plus cooling

oil, for greasing
7 ounces curly kale, stems removed, cut
    into large pieces
scant ½ cup cashews
2 tablespoons nutritional yeast flakes
    or 1 teaspoon garlic powder
1 small onion, roughly chopped
½ teaspoon turmeric
2 tablespoons apple cider vinegar
1 teaspoon sea salt

Savory Onion & Kale Chips

These healthy kale chips have a taste of cheese, but are, in fact, dairy-free—the flavor comes from using nutritional yeast flakes. Adding turmeric to the mix creates a golden glaze to the kale and it contains cancer-protective curcumin.

1 Heat the oven to 350°F and lightly grease 2 cookie sheets. Put the kale in a large bowl. Put the remaining ingredients into a blender or food processor and process to create a thick sauce. You might need to add 1 to 2 tablespoons water to thin the mixture.

2 Pour the mixture over the kale and use your hands to massage the sauce into the kale leaves so they are thoroughly coated. Arrange the kale, spaced apart, on the cookie sheets.

3 Bake 15 to 20 minutes, turning twice during cooking to make sure they become crisp. Remove the cookie sheets from the oven and leave the chips to cool before serving. (Store in an airtight container up to 3 days.)

NUTRITIONAL INFORMATION PER SERVING
Protein 3.6g, **Carbohydrates** 3.1g of which sugars 1.1g, **Fat** 4.2g of which saturates 0.8g, **Calories** 64

HEALTH BENEFITS
The nutritional yeast flakes are a good source of B vitamins. Kale contains cancer-protective nutrients, particularly glucosinolates, which are converted into isothiocyanates in the body, and have been shown to protect against bladder, breast, colon, ovary and prostate cancers. Kale also contains flavonoids, including kaempferol and quercetin, which possess important antioxidant and anti-inflammatory benefits helping lower inflammation and oxidative stress.

Spiced Flatbreads

Middle Eastern baked flatbreads make a perfect accompaniment to curries, soups and stews. Lightly spiced with cumin, these have the added health benefits of including turmeric, too.

1 Toast the cumin seeds in a dry skillet over medium heat until fragrant. Grind using a mortar and pestle. Put the yeast and honey in a measuring jug with ⅔ cup lukewarm water and stir to dissolve. Leave 10 minutes, or until frothy.

2 Sift the flours, turmeric, salt and cumin into a large bowl. Gradually pour in the yeast mixture. Add ⅔ cup lukewarm water and the olive oil, and mix to form a soft dough. Knead 5 minutes, or until smooth.

3 Put the dough in a greased bowl and cover with plastic wrap. Leave 1 hour, or until it doubles in size. Heat the oven to 425°F.

4 Divide the dough into 4 equal pieces. Roll each into an oval shape ¾ inch thick. Brush with a little water and sprinkle with sesame seeds. Bake direct on the oven shelf 7 to 10 minutes until puffed up. Transfer to a wire rack to cool slightly, then serve warm, or leave to cool completely. (Store, wrapped, in the refrigerator up to 3 days or freeze 1 month.)

MAKES 4

SERVES 8

PREPARATION TIME 25 minutes, plus 1¼ hours rising

COOKING TIME 10 minutes, plus cooling

1 tablespoon cumin seeds

2 envelopes (¼-oz.) active dry yeast

1 tablespoon raw honey

2 cups white bread flour

2 cups plus 1 tablespoon wholewheat bread flour

2 teaspoons turmeric

1 teaspoon salt

2 tablespoons olive oil, plus extra for greasing

1 tablespoon sesame seeds

NUTRITIONAL INFORMATION PER SERVING (½ FLATBREAD)
Protein 16.1g, **Carbohydrates** 86.7g of which sugars 6.5g, **Fat** 9.2g of which saturates 1.4g, **Calories** 493

HEALTH BENEFITS
The combination of wholewheat and white bread flours increases the nutritional profile and soluble fiber of the flatbreads. Turmeric contains curcumin, which possesses anti-inflammatory properties and is also cancer-protective.

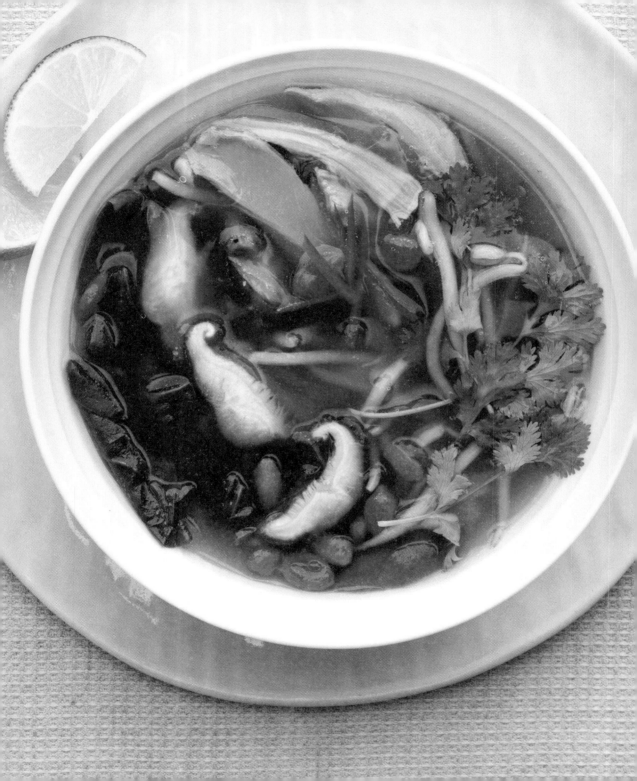

Supporting Your Body Through Treatment

Whether in combination with conventional cancer treatment or alone, good nutrition can help enhance your healing. A healthier diet might also alleviate some of the common side effects of the disease and/or the treatment. Incorporating certain key foods and herbs in your meals can assist you through your treatment and help your recovery. In this chapter you will find recipes designed to counter the symptoms of nausea, a loss of appetite, weight loss, low immune function, fatigue and digestive problems. Boost your energy with our Wheatgrass Energizer, snack on our Ginger, Almond & Chocolate Cookies to help manage nausea or support your immune health with our delicious Noodle, Shallot & Shiitake Salad.

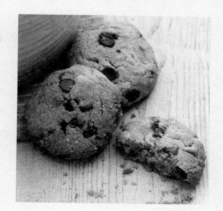

Opposite: Chicken-Ginger Miso Soup (page 147)
Above: Ginger, Almond & Chocolate Cookies (page 141)

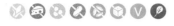

Ginger Vegetable Juice ▶

SERVES 2, 1 cup each
PREPARATION TIME 5 minutes

2 carrots
½ cucumber
2 celery sticks
1 lemon, peeled
3 apples
¾-inch piece of fresh gingerroot
ice cubes, to serve (optional)

1 Put all the ingredients through an electric juicer. Mix well and serve over ice, if you like. Drink immediately.

NUTRITIONAL INFORMATION PER SERVING
Protein 2g, **Carbohydrates** 19g of which sugars 18.9g,
Fat 0.6g of which saturates 0.1g, **Calories** 91

HEALTH BENEFITS
Cucumber is an excellent hydrator and contains lignans, which might be effective against certain types of cancers. The minerals potassium and sodium are present in celery and are important for regulating fluid balance.

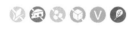

Gazpacho Smoothie

SERVES 1, 1 cup
PREPARATION TIME 5 minutes

3 vine-ripened tomatoes
½ cucumber
1 tablespoon chopped cilantro leaves
½ garlic clove, chopped
1 dash cayenne pepper, or to taste
¼ teaspoon ground cumin
1 teaspoon flaxseed oil
1 tablespoon lime juice
1 ripe pear, peeled and chopped
1 tablespoon seeds or nuts, to serve

1 Put all the ingredients into a blender or food processor and process until smooth. Add a little water to thin, if necessary. Drink immediately or store in the refrigerator up to 1 day. Serve with 1 tablespoon seeds or nuts.

NUTRITIONAL INFORMATION PER SERVING
Protein 6.4g, **Carbohydrates** 23.6g of which sugars 21.8g,
Fat 12.4g of which saturates 1.7g, **Calories** 237

HEALTH BENEFITS
Keeping yourself hydrated and nourished is important in controlling feelings of nausea. This smoothie is rich in electrolytes—sodium and potassium—that can help settle the stomach and reenergize you.

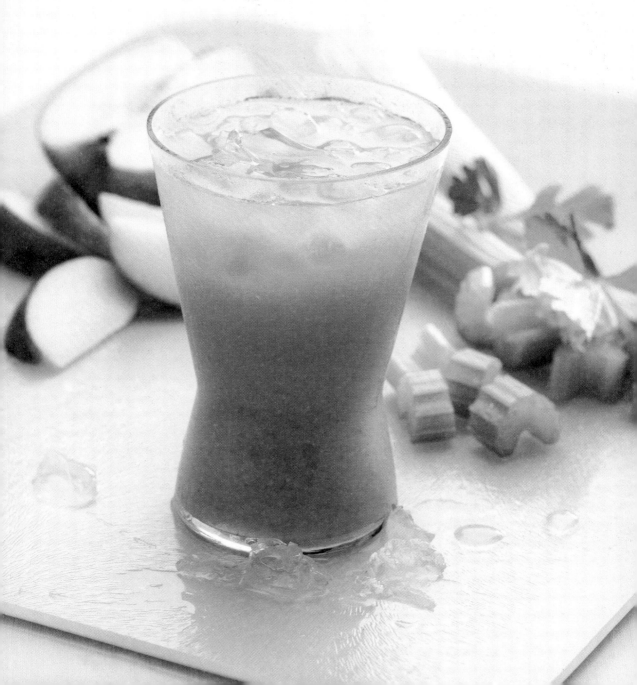

"Ginger is a remarkable natural aid to relieve digestive upsets and nausea."

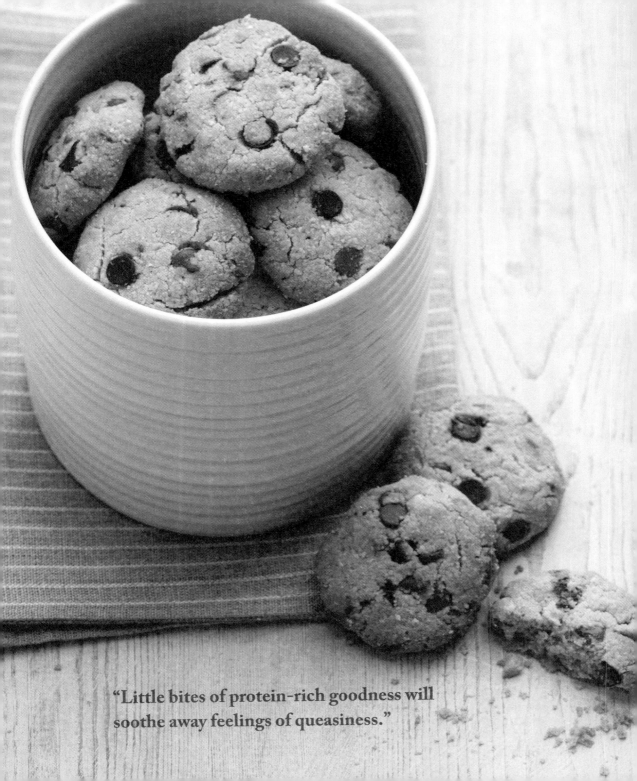

"Little bites of protein-rich goodness will soothe away feelings of queasiness."

Ginger, Almond & Chocolate Cookies

These soft cookies are ideal to snack on when you feel nauseous or your appetite is low. The perfect combination of ginger and chocolate makes them particularly tempting.

1 Heat the oven to 375°F and line a cookie sheet with baking parchment. Put the almonds in a bowl with the ground and fresh ginger, salt, baking soda and chocolate chips.

2 Mix together the remaining ingredients, then pour into the bowl and mix well.

3 Form the dough into walnut-size balls and press down lightly to form little cookies. Transfer to the cookie sheet and bake 12 to 15 minutes until lightly colored. Leave to cool on the cookie sheet 5 minutes, then transfer to a wire rack to cool completely before serving. (Store in an airtight container up to 1 week or freeze 1 month.)

MAKES 12
PREPARATION TIME 10 minutes
COOKING TIME 15 minutes, plus cooling

3 cups very finely ground blanched almonds
2 teaspoons ground ginger
¾-inch piece fresh gingerroot, peeled and finely grated
½ teaspoon sea salt
½ teaspoon baking soda
1 cup dark chocolate chips
3½ tablespoons almond nut butter or tahini
5 tablespoons plus 1 teaspoon butter, melted, or melted coconut oil
2¾ tablespoons raw honey

NUTRITIONAL INFORMATION PER COOKIE
Protein 6.9g, **Carbohydrates** 14.3g of which sugars 13.5g, **Fat** 27.2g of which saturates 9.7g, **Calories** 329

HEALTH BENEFITS
The high protein content of these cookies can help stabilize blood sugar levels, and this, too, can alleviate sickness. Almonds are a good source of magnesium for healthy nerve function, as well as containing manganese, copper and riboflavin (B2), which are energy-promoting nutrients.

Blueberry & Avocado Build-Up Shake

SERVES 2, 1 cup each

PREPARATION TIME 5 minutes

heaped ½ cup blanched almonds

1 tablespoon shelled hempseeds
or ground flaxseed

¼ cup whey vanilla protein powder
(optional)

1 ripe avocado, seeded and peeled

1 cup fresh or frozen blueberries, plus
extra to serve (optional)

1¼ cups coconut water or water

½ cup less 1 tablespoon coconut milk

½ cup less 1 tablespoon apple juice

2 teaspoons raw honey or manuka honey
(optional)

1 teaspoon slippery elm powder
(optional)

1 tablespoon coconut oil (optional)

2 teaspoons unsweetened cocoa powder
or cacao nibs

Soothing and creamy, thanks to the avocado and coconut milk, this revitalizing berry smoothie is packed with healthy fats, protein, vitamins and minerals. Make it in the morning and sip it throughout the day to help you maintain energy levels.

1 Put the almonds and seeds in a blender or food processor and process until finely ground.

2 Add the remaining ingredients and blend until light and creamy. Serve with more blueberries, if you like. (Store in the refrigerator up to 1 day.)

NUTRITIONAL INFORMATION PER SERVING
Protein 8.1g, **Carbohydrates** 31.8g of which sugars 19.9g, **Fat** 26.9g of which saturates 7.3g, **Calories** 399

HEALTH BENEFITS
Nutrient-dense avocados contain numerous anti-inflammatory compounds, including carotenoids, flavonoids, phytosterols and omega-3 and monounsaturated fats. The phytosterols, which constitute a major proportion of the fats in an avocado, help lower inflammation. Also included is oleic acid, which helps the body to absorb carotenoids and other fat-soluble nutrients. The unusual mix of anti-inflammatory and antioxidant nutrients found in avocados form the basis of their rich anticancer properties.

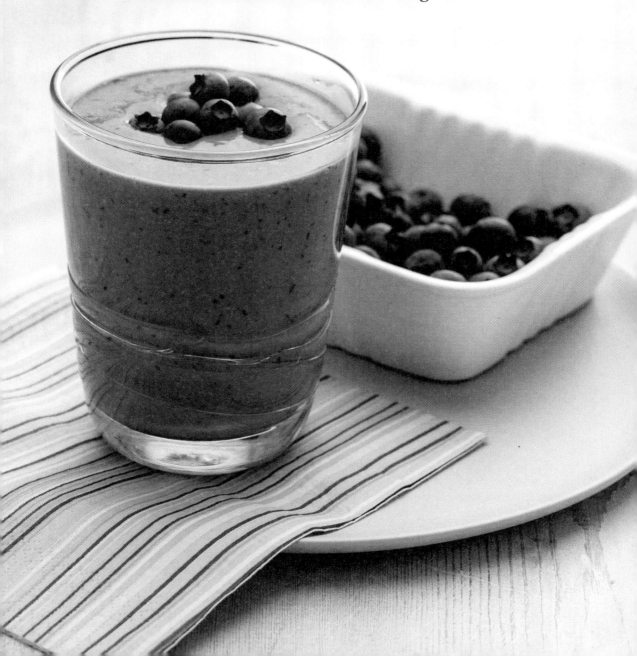

"Shakes and smoothies are ideal during treatment because they provide a nutritious meal in a glass."

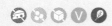

Almond & Pear Oatmeal

SERVES 4
PREPARATION TIME 5 minutes
COOKING TIME 10 minutes

2½ cups rolled oats or gluten-free oats
2 ripe pears, cored and chopped
3¾ cups almond or coconut milk
2 teaspoons cinnamon
¾ cup very finely ground blanched
   almonds
½ cup less 2 tablespoons oat cream
   or coconut cream
2 tablespoons ground flaxseed
1½ tablespoons chopped or slivered
   almonds

A warming oatmeal that is high in protein and healthy fats is a great way to start the day. Ground nuts and seeds provide protein, and the oatmeal is farther enriched with almond milk and oat cream. It makes a strengthening and appealing breakfast to help support your energy levels throughout the morning. The oatmeal can be made in advance and reheated in the morning with a little extra almond milk.

1 Put the oats, pears, milk and cinnamon into a saucepan. Bring gently to a boil, then lower the heat and simmer 6 to 7 minutes, stirring frequently, until the oats are soft and the mixture is thick.
2 Stir in the ground almonds, cream and flaxseed and beat well. Spoon into bowls and sprinkle the chopped almonds over the oatmeal to serve.

NUTRITIONAL INFORMATION PER SERVING
Protein 13.9g, **Carbohydrates** 54.4g of which sugars 21.4g, **Fat** 29.9g of which saturates 9.3g, **Calories** 542

HEALTH BENEFITS
Pears supply natural sweetness, while also having a low glycemic index. They are rich in soluble fiber, which supports blood sugar levels and digestive health. The addition of almonds to this dish provides a useful source of protein and the cancer-protective nutrients manganese and copper. Both of these minerals are important for the production of the key oxidative enzyme superoxide dismutase, which can help protect against damage caused by free radicals.

Cashew & Seed Bars

These raw bars are simple to prepare and provide valuable nutrients, as well as protein. Protein helps to support recovery during treatment and to maintain healthy muscle mass, and here it is present in the nuts, seeds and protein powder. The nuts also contain healthy fats and minerals, such as copper, manganese, calcium and magnesium.

MAKES 8

PREPARATION TIME 10 minutes,
    plus 1 hour chilling

1¼ cups cashews
3 tablespoons plus 1 teaspoon sesame
    seeds
1 tablespoon ground flaxseed
¼ cup vanilla whey protein powder
    or unsweetened shredded coconut
2 teaspoons green superfood powder
    of choice (optional)
heaped 1 cup ready-to-eat dried apricots
1 tablespoon apple juice, if needed

1 Line a cookie sheet with baking parchment. Put the nuts into a blender or food processor and process until coarsely ground. Tip into a bowl and add the sesame seeds and flaxseed.

2 Put the protein powder, green superfood powder, if using, and the apricots into a food processor and process to form a sticky dough. Add apple juice, if needed, to bring the mixture together. Add to the nut mixture and mix thoroughly with your hands to form a soft dough.

3 Put the dough onto the prepared cookie sheet and use your hands to press it out into a rectangle ¾ inch thick. Chill in the refrigerator 1 hour to firm slightly. Cut into 8 bars to serve. (Store in the refrigerator up to 1 week or freeze 1 month.)

NUTRITIONAL INFORMATION PER BAR
Protein 7.7g, **Carbohydrates** 13.4g of which sugars 9.5g, **Fat** 15.6g of which saturates 2.9g, **Calories** 225

HEALTH BENEFITS
Using the optional green superfood powder, such as spirulina, chlorella or barley grass, is an effective way to increase your intake of nutrients. Being rich in chlorophyll, these powders are particularly alkalizing and potent detoxifiers, too.

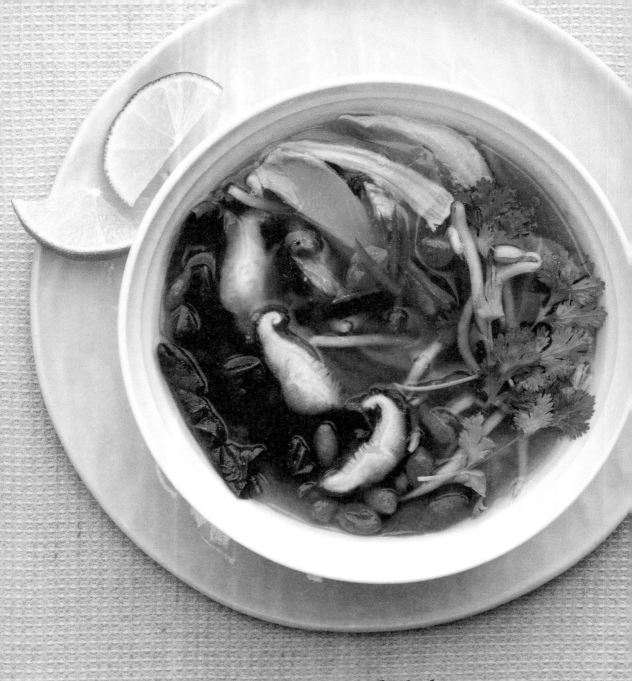

"You can't beat homemade chicken soup
for comfort and healing."

Chicken-Ginger Miso Soup

A homemade chicken soup retains all the goodness of the meat and vegetables, as well as possessing an appetizing and pronounced flavor. This one includes anti-inflammatory chili, garlic and ginger, and immune-supporting shiitake mushrooms. The soup can be frozen in batches, making it ideal to prepare during treatment.

SERVES 6

PREPARATION TIME 15 minutes

COOKING TIME 2 hours 20 minutes

1 chicken, 2¼ to 3 pounds
1 teaspoon black peppercorns
2½-inch piece fresh gingerroot, peeled and sliced
1 large onion, cut into wedges
4 garlic cloves, crushed
2 tablespoons Thai fish sauce, or to taste
1 handful spinach leaves or 1 bok choy
3⅓ cups beansprouts or sprouted mung beans
1 red onion, finely chopped
1 red chili, seeded and finely sliced lengthwise (optional)
6 shiitake mushrooms, sliced
3 tablespoons goji berries (optional)
a squeeze lime juice
1 tablespoon white sweet miso paste
leaves from 1 bunch cilantro

1 First make the stock. Put the chicken into a large saucepan and cover with 3 quarts water. Add the peppercorns, half the ginger, the onion and 2 garlic cloves and bring to a boil. Reduce to a simmer and add the fish sauce. Simmer 1 hour, or until the meat is tender.

2 Lift out the chicken, then shred the meat. Return the bones to the stock and simmer 1 hour longer. Strain the stock and reserve. Discard the vegetables and bones.

3 Bring the stock to a boil, then simmer 10 minutes. Add the remaining ginger and the chicken, spinach, beansprouts, red onion, chili, if using, the remaining garlic and the mushrooms. Simmer 2 to 3 minutes longer to heat through, then add the goji berries, if using, the lime juice, miso and cilantro. Add more fish sauce to taste, if needed. Stir for 1 minute, then serve. (Store in the refrigerator up to 3 days or freeze 1 month.)

NUTRITIONAL INFORMATION PER SERVING

Protein 34.7g, **Carbohydrates** 10.2g of which sugars 7.7g, **Fat** 24g of which saturates 6.4g, **Calories** 396

HEALTH BENEFITS

Chicken is an excellent source of easily digestible protein and of the cancer-protective B vitamin, niacin, as well as selenium. Selenium has been shown to induce DNA repair and synthesis in damaged cells, to inhibit the proliferation of cancer cells and to induce cell death.

Noodle, Shallot & Shiitake Salad

SERVES 4

PREPARATION TIME 20 minutes, plus 15 minutes soaking

COOKING TIME 30 minutes

12 small shallots, cut in half if large
1 tablespoon olive oil
1 tablespoon balsamic vinegar
½ ounce dulse
14 ounces rice or kelp noodles
12 asparagus spears
1 red bell pepper, seeded and cut into matchstick strips
8 shiitake mushrooms, sliced
freshly ground black pepper

Dressing

2 tablespoons each sesame oil and olive oil
3 tablespoons each tamari and balsamic vinegar
a pinch crushed chilies (optional)
2 teaspoons raw honey
1 garlic clove, crushed
½-inch piece fresh gingerroot, grated
1 handful cilantro leaves, chopped

Rice noodles are perfect for using with this rich balsamic dressing, because they readily absorb the strong flavors. Combined with shiitake mushrooms, asparagus and shallots, they make a satisfying salad. The light-tasting sea vegetable, dulse, is added for its mineral-rich qualities. Just a small handful is sufficient, as it swells once soaked. For protein, add a little cooked and flaked salmon or trout.

1 Heat the oven to 350°F. Put the shallots in a roasting pan and drizzle with the oil and vinegar. Roast 30 minutes, or until golden. Meanwhile, soak the dulse 15 minutes, then drain and chop.

2 Mix together all the dressing ingredients. Soak the noodles 3 minutes, or according to the package directions, then drain and put into a large bowl.

3 Cut the asparagus diagonally into ¾-inch pieces, then put it into a steamer and steam over high heat 1 minute, or until just tender. Drain and refresh in cold water, then drain again. Put the asparagus and shallots into the bowl and add the remaining ingredients. Pour the dressing over and toss to coat. Season with pepper, then serve. (Store, without dressing, in the refrigerator up to 3 days.)

NUTRITIONAL INFORMATION PER SERVING
Protein 7g, **Carbohydrates** 73.5g of which sugars 7.1g, **Fat** 11.7g of which saturates 1.7g, **Calories** 462

HEALTH BENEFITS
Shiitake mushrooms are a powerful immunomodulator, enhancing the function of immune cells in recognizing and destroying cancer cells. Sea vegetables—dulse and the optional kelp noodles—are useful sources of iodine, important in the prevention of breast cancer.

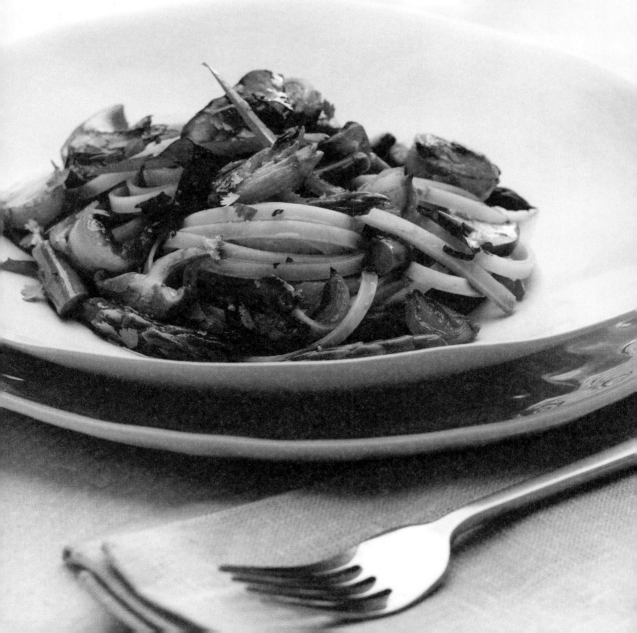

"Benefit from the immune-enhancing properties of sea vegetables and shiitake mushrooms."

"Relieve flagging energy levels with the benefits of beet, cucumber and apple."

Wheatgrass Energizer

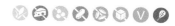

1 Put all the ingredients through an electric juicer. Serve over ice, if you like. Drink immediately.

SERVES 1, 1 cup
PREPARATION TIME: 5 minutes

1 green apple
1 celery stick
1 handful spinach
1 bunch wheatgrass or 1 cube frozen
  wheatgrass
½ lemon
ice cubes, to serve (optional)

NUTRITIONAL INFORMATION PER SERVING
Protein 4.2g, **Carbohydrates** 9.6g of which sugars 9.1g,
Fat 0.6g of which saturates 0.1g, **Calories** 61

HEALTH BENEFITS
Wheatgrass contains at least thirteen vitamins (including antioxidants and B12),
minerals and trace elements, including selenium. It is also a complete source of amino
acids (protein building blocks). Chlorophyll has almost the same molecular structure
as hemoglobin and helps to oxygenate the body.

◂ Stamina-Boosting Beet Juice

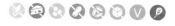

1 Put all the ingredients through an electric juicer. Stir well and drink immediately.

SERVES 1, 1 cup
PREPARATION TIME 5 minutes

2 apples
1 raw beet (about 5 ounces)
½ cucumber
½ lemon, peeled

NUTRITIONAL INFORMATION PER SERVING
Protein 4.3g, **Carbohydrates** 27.2g of which sugars 26.9g,
Fat 0.6g of which saturates 0g, **Calories** 133

HEALTH BENEFITS
Studies have shown beets can increase levels of nitric oxide in the body, which affects
blood flow, hormone levels and cell signaling.

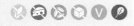

SERVES 4
PREPARATION TIME 10 minutes
COOKING TIME 4 minutes

2 scallions
½ ripe avocado, seeded and peeled
2 ripe pears, cored
¾ cucumber
1 celery stick
2 tablespoons lemon juice
1 tablespoon chopped mint leaves,
   plus extra to serve
2 ounces baby spinach leaves
   or watercress
2 teaspoons ground cumin
a pinch cayenne pepper
a pinch sea salt
1 tablespoon tamari
1 cup plus 2 tablespoons coconut water,
   water or vegetable stock
freshly ground black pepper
sliced scallion, to serve

Green Energy Soup

The perfect meal for when you feel too tired to cook: a light, nurturing, super-quick soup that can be served warm or cold. Pears provide natural sweetness to offset the strong flavor of the nutrient-rich spinach. Also included are "hydrating" vegetables—rich in electrolytes, especially potassium—to keep the body's fluids balanced.

1 Put all the ingredients into a blender or food processor and process until smooth. If serving warm, pour the soup into a saucepan and gently warm through 3 to 4 minutes, stirring occasionally.
2 Spoon into bowls and serve sprinkled with chopped mint and scallion and season with pepper. (Store in the refrigerator 1 day.)

NUTRITIONAL INFORMATION PER SERVING
Protein 1.3g, **Carbohydrates** 8.1g of which sugars 8g, **Fat** 2.9g of which saturates 0.5g, **Calories** 63

HEALTH BENEFITS
Spinach is a rich source of folic acid and also contains vitamin B6. Folic acid, plus B6 and methionine, can help the body to protect and repair DNA, and, therefore, these nutrients play an important role in inhibiting cancer development. B vitamins are also needed for energy production. The soup also contains phytonutrients and some unique anticancer carotenoids, called epoxyxanthophylls.

Chicken Liver Salad with Cider Vinegar Dressing

Nutrient-rich greens contrast with sweet apple and crunchy walnuts in this salad to serve with chicken livers —brought together with a tangy dressing. Choose organic liver, if you can, as it provides the greatest health benefits.

SERVES 4
PREPARATION TIME 10 minutes
COOKING TIME 10 minutes

scant 1 cup walnut pieces or pecans
14 ounces chicken livers
1 large head romaine lettuce or other lettuce
2 small handfuls watercress
1 apple, diced
2 celery sticks, finely diced
2 tablespoons chopped parsley leaves
1 tablespoon olive oil, ghee or coconut oil
sea salt and freshly ground black pepper

Cider vinegar dressing
2 tablespoons apple cider vinegar
1 teaspoon Dijon mustard
5 tablespoons olive oil

1 Lightly toast the walnuts in a dry skillet over medium heat 1 minute, stirring, then chop them roughly. Set aside. Remove the sinew from the livers, and cut the livers in half, if large. Season with salt and pepper and set aside.

2 Tear the lettuce and watercress and put it into a bowl with the apple, celery and parsley. Whisk the dressing ingredients together and season. Spoon 1 to 2 tablespoons over the leaves and toss to lightly coat. Add the walnuts and toss lightly. Divide among 4 plates.

3 Heat the olive oil in a large, heavy-bottomed skillet over medium heat. Fry the livers 3 to 4 minutes on each side until brown and just cooked through to the middle. Remove from the heat and arrange on the salad leaves.

4 Put the remaining dressing in the pan. Allow it to bubble a few seconds, then drizzle over the salad and serve. (Store, without dressing, in the refrigerator up to 1 day.)

NUTRITIONAL INFORMATION PER SERVING
Protein 22.9g, **Carbohydrates** 4.5g of which sugars 4.4g, **Fat** 33.6g of which saturates 6.3g, **Calories** 412

HEALTH BENEFITS
Chicken liver is an exceptionally nutrient-dense food, representing an excellent source of zinc, vitamins B12 and A, copper, selenium and protein, and a good source of iron—especially important for relieving fatigue and energizing the body.

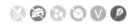

Coconut-Cocoa Booster

SERVES 2
PREPARATION TIME 5 minutes

2 teaspoons unsweetened cocoa powder
  or raw cacao powder, or to taste
1 teaspoon maca powder
1 tablespoon ground flaxseed
1 cup plus 2 tablespoons coconut milk
1 cup plus 2 tablespoons coconut water
  or water
2 teaspoons coconut oil (optional)
1 banana
2 tablespoons seeds or nuts, to serve

1 Put all the ingredients into a blender or food processor and process until smooth. Drink immediately or store in the refrigerator up to 1 day. To serve hot, heat the blended drink gently in a saucepan until hot but not boiling. Serve each drink with 1 tablespoon seeds or nuts.

NUTRITIONAL INFORMATION PER SERVING
Protein 4.5g, **Carbohydrates** 28g of which sugars 16g,
Fat 7.3g of which saturates 3.4g, **Calories** 194

HEALTH BENEFITS
Maca is a Peruvian root that can be bought in powdered form. It has traditionally been used to support the body in times of stress. (Maca can also be added to baking recipes.)

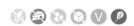

Chia-Papaya Pudding▶

SERVES 2
PREPARATION TIME 5 minutes,
  plus 15 minutes soaking

4 tablespoons chia seeds
6 pitted dried dates
⅔ cup cashews
a pinch cinnamon
a pinch sea salt
1 ripe papaya, peeled, seeded and sliced
2 tablespoons flaked coconut

1 Soak the chia seeds in water 15 minutes. Put all the ingredients, except the papaya and coconut, into a blender or food processor with 2 cups plus 2 tablespoons water and process until smooth. Serve topped with the papaya and coconut. (Store in the refrigerator up to 1 day.)

NUTRITIONAL INFORMATION PER SERVING
Protein 7.5g, **Carbohydrates** 18.1g of which sugars 6.3g,
Fat 20.2g of which saturates 6.6g, **Calories** 281

HEALTH BENEFITS
Chia seeds are rich in omega-3 and easily digestible protein and fiber. Papaya contains protective antioxidants and the digestive enzyme, papain.

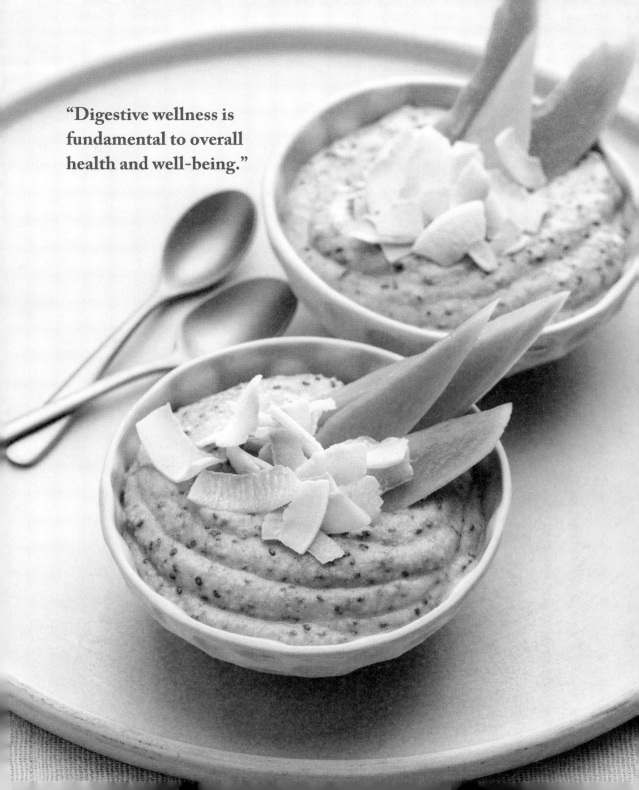

"Digestive wellness is fundamental to overall health and well-being."

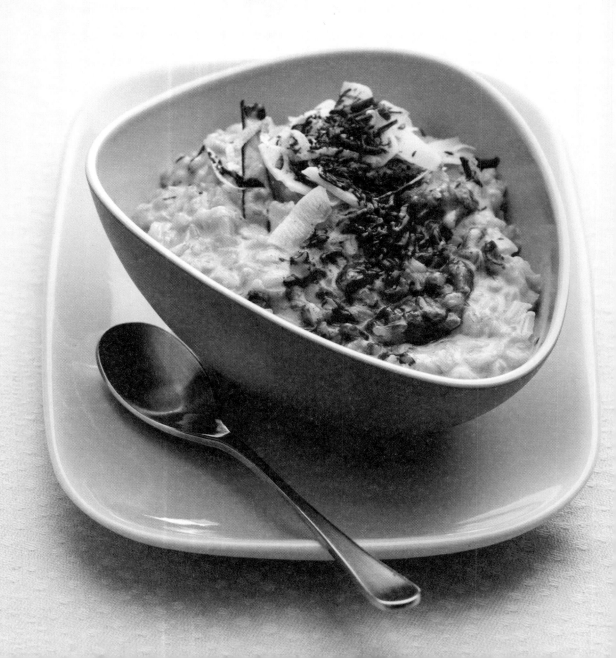

"Richly flavored, yet beautifully soothing for the digestion."

Coconut Rice Pudding

Toasting the rice in the butter gives it a rich nuttiness, which is complemented by the caramel flavor of the molasses. Adding the dash of molasses gives sweetness to the dessert, as well as providing potassium, calcium and iron. B vitamins, soluble fiber and slow-releasing complex carbohydrate are also present.

1 Heat the butter in a large saucepan over medium heat and add the rice. Stir to coat it in the butter 2 to 3 minutes to create a nutty flavor.

2 Pour in the coconut milk, vanilla, cinnamon stick and lemon zest and juice. Bring to a boil, then lower the heat and simmer 30 minutes, stirring occasionally.

3 Add the molasses, flaxseed, coconut flakes and most of the chocolate and cook 10 to 15 minutes longer, stirring occasionally. The rice should be very tender and most of the liquid absorbed. Remove the pan from the heat and leave the rice to stand, covered, 5 minutes. Serve warm or chilled, and sprinkle the remaining chocolate on top with a few coconut flakes and lemon zest, if you like. (You can add all the chocolate at the beginning of step 3, if you prefer.) (Store in the refrigerator up to 2 days.)

SERVES 6
PREPARATION TIME 5 minutes
COOKING TIME 50 minutes,
   plus 5 minutes standing

2 tablespoons butter or coconut oil
1¾ cups long-grain brown rice
5½ cups coconut milk
1 teaspoon vanilla extract
1 cinnamon stick, broken in half
zest and juice of 1 lemon, plus extra zest
   to serve (optional)
1 tablespoon molasses
1 tablespoon ground flaxseed
½ cup coconut flakes, plus extra to serve
   (optional)
¾ ounce dark chocolate (at least 75%
   cocoa solids), grated, or 1 tablespoon
   cacao nibs

NUTRITIONAL INFORMATION PER SERVING
Protein 5.4g, **Carbohydrates** 57.7g of which sugars 13.8g, **Fat** 9.9g of which saturates 6.5g, **Calories** 342

HEALTH BENEFITS
The soluble fiber in the rice is gentle on the digestive system and useful for relieving diarrhea and constipation. Coconut milk and coconut oil provide a source of lauric acid for immune health and caprylic acid to support the gut.

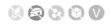

Italian Crackers & Bean Dip

SERVES 6
PREPARATION TIME 15 minutes
COOKING TIME 45 minutes,
  plus cooling

1½ cups flaxseeds
⅓ cup almonds
1 red bell pepper, seeded and chopped
1 tomato, chopped
1 egg
zest and juice of ½ lemon
½ cup pitted ripe olives
1 tablespoon chopped basil leaves
sea salt and freshly ground black pepper

Curried bean dip
1 can (15-oz.) cannellini beans, drained
  and rinsed
1 teaspoon turmeric
2 garlic cloves
½ teaspoon ground cumin
1 tablespoon lemon juice
about 2 tablespoons olive oil
1 tablespoon chopped parsley leaves

Baking these crackers in a low oven preserves their omega-3 content. Serve them as a snack or for a light meal with the dip, which contains cancer-protective turmeric.

1 Heat the oven to 300°F and line a cookie sheet with baking parchment. Grind the flaxseeds and almonds in a food processor until fine. Add the red pepper and tomato, and process until combined.

2 Add the egg and lemon zest and juice, then season with salt and pepper. Process to form a thick dough. Briefly pulse in the olives and stir in the basil.

3 Using a spatula and damp hands, spread the mixture onto the cookie sheet ¼ inch thick, then shape into a square. Score to make individual crackers. Bake 40 to 45 minutes until lightly colored and crisp.

4 Put all the ingredients for the curried bean dip into a food processor and season lightly. Process until smooth. Add a little extra oil, if needed.

5 Break the flaxseed mixture into individual crackers along the score lines and leave to cool on a wire rack. Serve with the dip. (Store the crackers in an airtight container up to 4 days. Store the dip in the refrigerator up to 3 days.)

NUTRITIONAL INFORMATION PER SERVING OF CRACKERS
Protein 3.3g, **Carbohydrates** 4.4g of which sugars 1.1g, **Fat** 7.6g of which saturates 0.8g, **Calories** 95

NUTRITIONAL INFORMATION PER SERVING OF DIP
Protein 2.4g, **Carbohydrates** 4.7g of which sugars 0.5g, **Fat** 3.3g of which saturates 0.5g, **Calories** 57

HEALTH BENEFITS
The fiber content helps support overall digestive health, which is particularly important in reducing the risk of bowel cancer.

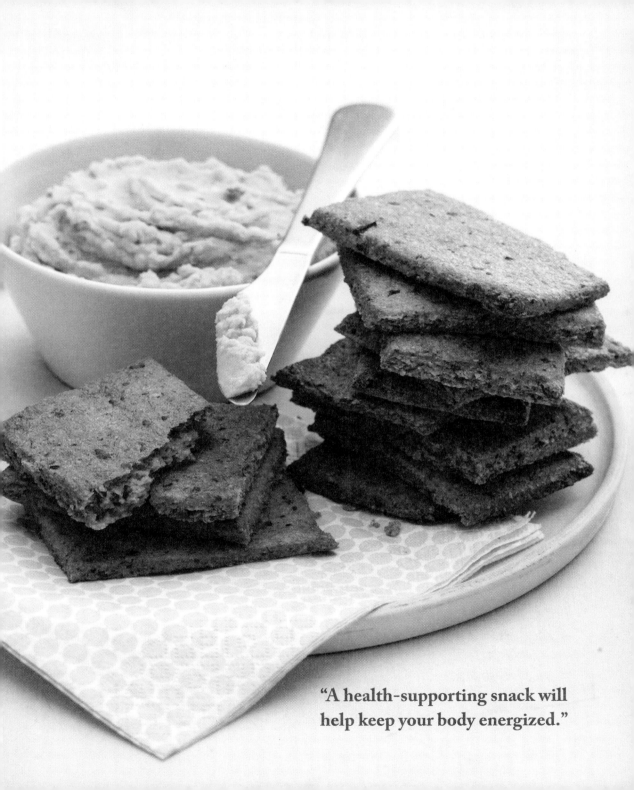

"A health-supporting snack will help keep your body energized."

Index

alcohol 43
Almond-Citrus Cake 125
Almond & Pear Oatmeal 144
angiogenesis 13
antioxidants 15
appetite: loss of 30–1
Apple, Walnut & Pistachio Crumble 122
Asian Turkey Patties with Dipping Sauce 75
Avocado & Lime Mousse 129

Baked Lemon Cheesecake 123
Balsamic-Braised Duck 100
barbecuing 22
Bell Pepper Bisque with Chili Cream 74
Blueberry & Avocado Build-Up Shake 142
bones: healthy 42–3
Brazil Nut Cream Smoothie 53
Broccoli & Cashew Soup 68

caffeine 43
carbohydrates 17
Cashew & Seed Bars 145
Celery Root, Apple & Fennel Rémoulade 88
cell division 14
Chia-Papaya Pudding 154
Chicken & Cashew Stir-Fry 94
Chicken-Ginger Miso Soup 147
Chicken Liver Salad with Cider Vinegar Dressing 153
Chocolate & Beet Bars 133
Coconut-Cocoa Booster 154
Coconut- & Lime-Baked Sardines 81
Coconut Rice Pudding 157
condiments: natural 39–40
constipation 33
Creamy Cauliflower Soup 72

dairy products 20; alternatives 42–3
Date & Lucuma Cocoa Bars 60
diarrhea 33
digestion 32, 38
Digestive Healer 52

fatigue 30
fats 12, 17, 19, 21
Flaxseed, Apricot & Cinnamon Muffins 59
free radicals 15
fruit 16, 17, 18

Garlic & Bean Soup with Pesto 71
Gazpacho Smoothie 138
genes 14
Ginger, Almond & Chocolate Cookies 141
Ginger & Umeboshi Chicken 97
Ginger Vegetable Juice 138
glycemic index (GI) 13
glycemic load (GL) 13
Gooey Chocolate & Raspberry Pudding 120
Green Elixir 52
Green Energy Soup 152
Green Hemp Shake 51
Green Tea Ice Cream 126

healthy eating 16–23, 36–41
Hempseed & Nut Burgers 116
herbs 17, 20
Hoisin Tempeh Skewers 84
hormonal imbalances 14

inflammation 12, 13
insulin resistance 14
Italian Crackers & Bean Dip 158

Japanese Lamb Burgers with Wasabi Mayo 78

Legumes 19

Matcha & Mango Shake 51
Matcha Tea & Banana Bread 130
meat 20, 22
menu plans 46–7
Miso-Glazed Salmon 108
Mixed Sea Vegetable & Cucumber Salad 90
Mixed Seafood Pie 109
Mixed Seed Granola 56
mouth ulcers 31–2
nausea 31
Noodle, Shallot & Shiitake Salad 148
nutrients 24–9

obesity 14
omega-3 fatty acids 12
oral thrush 31–2
organic food 16, 42

Pan-Fried Squid with Red Cabbage & Walnuts 83
Persian Quinoa Omega Bowl 117

processed meats 22
proteins 16–17, 18

Redbush Apricot Smoothie 53
refined grains 21
Roasted Sea Bass with Olives & Tomatoes 103
Roasted Tempeh with Pipérade Sauce 110

Salmon with Sauce Vierge 104
salt 22
Sardines with Roasted Tomatoes 65
Savory Onion & Kale Chips 134
Sicilian Shrimp 82
smell, sense of 31
soy products 21, 44–5
Spaghetti with Lemon & Broccoli 114
Spanish Baked Eggs 63
Spiced Flatbreads 135
spices 17, 20
Stamina-Boosting Beet Juice 151
Star Anise-Poached Plums with Ginger-Nut Cream 55
stress 15
sugars 13, 21, 41
Super-Berry Yogurt Sorbet 126
Super-Greens Salad with Chicken 77
supplements 45
swallowing problems 31–2
sweeteners 41

Tamarind-Spiced Mackerel 107
taste, sense of 31
trans-fats 12, 21
Turkey & Pistachio Korma 98
Turkish Breakfast 64

vegans 44
vegetables 16, 17, 18
vegetarians 44
Venison with Zesty Gremolata 101

Warm Eggplant, Roots & Chickpea Salad 113
Warm Lentil & Bean Salad 91
water 22–3
weight 34–5
Wheatgrass Energizer 151
whole grains 19
Wilted Kale Salad with Toasted Seeds 87